Suicide Prevention and New Technologies

Suicide Prevention and New Technologies

Evidence Based Practice

Edited by

Brian L. Mishara
Université du Québec à Montréal, Montreal, Quebec, Canada

and

Ad J. F. M. Kerkhof
VU University, Amsterdam, The Netherlands

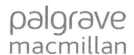

palgrave
macmillan

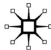
First published 2013 by
PALGRAVE MACMILLAN

Palgrave Macmillan in the UK is an imprint of Macmillan Publishers Limited,
registered in England, company number 785998, of Houndmills, Basingstoke,
Hampshire RG21 6XS.

Palgrave Macmillan in the US is a division of St Martin's Press LLC,
175 Fifth Avenue, New York, NY 10010.

Palgrave Macmillan is the global academic imprint of the above companies
and has companies and representatives throughout the world.

Palgrave® and Macmillan® are registered trademarks in the United States,
the United Kingdom, Europe and other countries

ISBN: 978–1–137–35168–5 hardback
ISBN: 978–1–137–35171–5 paperback

This book is printed on paper suitable for recycling and made from fully
managed and sustained forest sources. Logging, pulping and manufacturing
processes are expected to conform to the environmental regulations of the
country of origin.

A catalogue record for this book is available from the British Library.

A catalog record for this book is available from the Library of Congress.

Contents

v

List of Tables

List of Figures

Preface: The Future of Suicide Prevention at Our Doorstep

New technologies have entered the field of suicide prevention with great expectations for the future, despite a relatively slow start. The Internet, mobile phones and computer self-help programmes have a strong potential to reach, support and help suicidal people, their families, teachers, caregivers and bereaved survivors. Worldwide the use of new technologies is beginning to be embraced by volunteers and professionals, by crisis lines, suicide prevention centres, mental health centres, researchers and politicians. This has created a wave of hope that new, better and cheaper services will soon be available to effectively reach and help vulnerable people and prevent suicides. The potential of helping vulnerable people who do not use conventional mental health services and people in regions with limited psychiatric facilities is appealing.

But is all this enthusiasm justified? Do new technologies really help reach those people who most need support? Similar concerns were raised when telephone helpline services came into operation over 50 years ago. This question proved difficult to answer, and many decades of research were needed to finally conclude that telephonic helplines do help callers, but their impact on suicide rates is not easy to demonstrate. Similar questions are to be answered in the near future: Do we really reach people at risk of suicide when offering Internet-based interventions, and do we help them? Can smartphone applications prevent repeated suicide attempts? Are lives really saved by using new technologies? Does using new technologies actually reduce costs and provide better services when compared to traditional approaches? The quest for answers to these questions constitutes a priority research agenda as we increasingly invest in suicide prevention using new technologies. In the following section we briefly introduce the main uses of new technologies that are presented in this book.

Obtaining information on suicide and suicide prevention is now easy through efficient search engines and helpful links. The Internet has accelerated the spread of knowledge to the general public, including general information, warning signs for suicide, risk factors, articles and videos on suicide and suicide prevention, and treatment recommendations. Suicide prevention organizations post valuable information for the public, for journalists, for suicidal people, their relatives, caregivers, for the bereaved survivors, for gatekeepers and for researchers. All this has undoubtedly increased the level of awareness in society of suicide as a public health problem. Anyone with an Internet connection can find almost anything the person wants to know about suicide. Relatives, who are concerned about depressive or suicidal behaviour of a loved one, can look for information and guidance about how to assess the situation and persuade their relative to get help. This "gatekeeper" function of relatives has probably been strengthened enormously by access to the Internet.

Suicidal people also surf the Internet for information about how to commit suicide. One can easily find the many websites that offer explicit information about suicide methods. Just type in Google: how to commit suicide? You will find a lot of nonsense, sick humour, as well as explicit, but not always reliable, information about the pros and cons of particular methods, including their speed, how to use the method and the likely amount of pain associated with it. There is no control of the accuracy of Internet content and, as is discussed in Chapter 1 by Mishara and Côté and Chapter 13 by Kerkhof and Mishara, there are both risks and benefits of the mass of information on suicide now available on the Internet.

There are huge numbers of discussion forums or platforms for exchange of opinions and experiences and chat forums where suicide related issues are posted and discussed. In Chapter 2, Thoër reviews the nature of interactions on these group platforms. Benefits and dangers of such discussion groups are also described in Chapter 1 (Mishara and Côté). There are sites using group text messaging forums for specific groups, such as the platforms for the bereaved, described in Chapter 11 by Krysinska and Andriessen, sometimes associated with online memorials. These platforms for the bereaved focus on mutual support and recognition of each other's experiences.

Many new developments provide for interactive exchanges with suicide prevention organizations, such as the National Suicide Prevention Lifeline in the United States (Chapter 9 by Murphy), and 113Online in the Netherlands (Chapter 10 by Mokkenstorm and colleagues). These organizations provide some combination of: immediate assistance in crisis, online emotional support by telephone, text messaging services, self-testing or interactive assessment, guidance for self-help interventions, professional crisis counselling and immediate referral to acute psychiatric services if deemed necessary and possible. Services mostly are free of charge, available 24 hours every day, anonymous and easily accessible. A thorough review of emotional support by crisis-chat is presented in Chapter 8 by Drexler.

The possibility of identifying, locating and intervening with suicidal persons, even against the callers' will, poses serious ethical questions. Should we proactively intervene, justifying the intervention by the rationale that protection of life is more important than any potential intrusion into privacy? Ethical dilemmas in the use of new technologies in suicide preventions are discussed in Chapter 5 by Mishara and Weisstub and in the concluding chapter (Chapter 13).

From the e-mental health perspective, many studies have demonstrated the effectiveness of guided or unguided web-based self-help for mental disorders, including depression, panic disorder, general anxiety disorder, social phobia and problem drinking. Chapter 3 by Hatcher presents an overview of e-therapies in suicide prevention. In this book, we also present an entirely autonomous computer program on a textual learning platform that people can access as a cognitive behavioural self-help therapy programme for worrisome suicide ideation (Chapter 4 by Kerkhof and colleagues).

There is also e-learning for volunteers and professionals stemming from the world of telemedicine and telecare, a fast growing body of one-way or interactive video learning programmes on the Internet. E-learning modules for improving knowledge, attitudes and skills in suicide prevention have been developed for use particularly in the education and training of professionals in mental health care. An example of e-learning modules for teachers and school counsellors to help them identify and refer adolescents at risk of suicide is provided in Chapter 6 by Ghoncheh and colleagues.

As an increasingly large proportion of people around the world now have smartphones, mobile phone applications may become an increasingly present therapeutic adjunct in the treatment of depressed, suicidal and self-harming patients. Smart phones can become an emergency tool with an automated safety plan available in the event of a suicidal crisis. Chapter 12 by Labelle and colleagues describes a comprehensive mobile phone application which can even send an emergency call to five members of the person's support network if distress levels demand rapid assistance, with geo-location of the caller as well as nearby emergency care facilities.

Recently, virtual reality programs with avatars or gaming programs have been developed for suicide prevention. In Chapter 7, Pommereau describes a programme where self-destructive teenagers create avatars or digital doubles of themselves, dress them up with realistic accessories, thereby expressing themselves as they see themselves in their inner world, including their emotional pain and misery. This technology has the promise of enabling more effective therapeutic interactions to deal with an adolescent's pain and misery, which would be more difficult to realize without the self-representations in digital avatars.

As is usually the case, when new prevention measures are first tried, research is lagging behind in evaluating the effects of these new technologies in suicide prevention. This means that we do not yet know which of these new initiatives work most effectively, under what conditions and whether they really help prevent suicides. Mishara and Côté provide a review of the theory and the meagre evidence we now have to justify practices (Chapter 1). In Chapter 13 a research agenda is presented and challenges for the development and use of new technologies are discussed.

This book presents the reader with a contemporary survey of new technologies and suicide prevention, developments, possibilities, dilemmas, current knowledge and concrete examples. This is a rapidly changing field. At the present time we have more questions than answers. Still, the excitement about the potential for suicide prevention is increasing exponentially, despite the numerous concerns. Please send us your comments and further thoughts on this group chat forum, as well as information to help us update this book for future editions: www.misharakerkhof.ca.

Notes on Contributors

Brian L. Mishara is Professor of Psychology and Director of the Centre for Research and Intervention on Suicide and Euthanasia (CRISE) at the Université du Québec in Montréal. He is Vice-Chairperson of the Trustees of Befrienders Worldwide, an organization of helplines and volunteer-based suicide prevention centres around the world. His publications, including six books in English and five in French in the areas of suicidology and gerontology, include research on the effectiveness of suicide prevention programmes, studies of how children develop an understanding of suicide, theories of the development of suicidality, ethical issues in research, euthanasia and "assisted suicide," and evaluations of helpline effectiveness. Professor Mishara was a founder of Suicide Action Montreal, the Montreal suicide prevention centre and the Quebec Association for Suicide Prevention. He was a past president of the International Association for Suicide Prevention (IASP) and the Canadian Association for Suicide Prevention. He also consults and conducts training for suicide prevention organizations internationally, including helplines that provide services over the Internet.

Ad J. F. M. Kerkhof is Professor of Clinical Psychology, Psychopathology and Suicide Prevention at the VU University in Amsterdam, The Netherlands. He has worked for over 30 years in suicide research, teaching and clinical work in suicide prevention. He has studied attitudes towards suicide, suicide in correctional facilities, train suicides, epidemiology of attempted suicide, online suicide prevention, self-help intervention for suicidal worrying, screening of suicidal adolescents, and implementation of practice guidelines for the assessment and treatment of suicidal behaviour. He developed training protocols in suicide prevention for mental health care professionals, gatekeepers and volunteers of crisis lines. He was editor in chief of *Crisis*, the scientific journal of the International Association for Suicide Prevention, and was one of the authors of the Dutch practice guidelines for the assessment and treatment of suicidal behaviour, in 2012 approved by the professional organizations in health care. Recently, he developed a cognitive behavioural treatment for suicidal worries, which has been tested in a randomized controlled trial using an online self-help treatment. He is on the board of directors of 113Online.

Karl Andriessen is a staff member at the Federation of Tele-Help Centres (Tele-Onthaal) in Flanders-Belgium where he facilitates suicide prevention and postvention training for staff members and volunteers. He is also a researcher at the Faculty of Psychology and Educational Sciences, KU Leuven – University of Leuven, Belgium. He is Co-Chair of the Special Interest Group on Suicide Bereavement and Postvention of the International Association for Suicide Prevention.

Louis-Philippe Côté is a doctoral candidate in the Psychology Department of the Université du Québec in Montreal. His doctoral dissertation research involves an empirical investigation of the effectiveness of different Internet chat intervention methods with suicidal persons.

Mary Drexler currently serves as part-time Executive Director for CONTACT USA, a network of crisis intervention centers across the nation. She has an extensive background in crisis intervention and suicide prevention. She worked for 11 years as a Crisis Center Director in Connecticut that served residents statewide. She has been in the social services field since 1979. She served three years as Crisis Division Chair on the Council of Delegates for the American Association of Suicidology and is also an ASIST trainer. She is also a private consultant, focusing primarily in the areas of suicide prevention and intervention. Mary also serves as the full-time Executive Director of the Connecticut Council on Problem Gambling (CCPG). She holds a masters degree in Social Work from the University of Connecticut School of Social Work.

Rezvan Ghoncheh is a doctoral candidate in the Departments of Clinical and Developmental Psychology at VU University Faculty of Psychology and Education, and EMGO+ Institute for Health Care Research. Her doctoral dissertation is on the development and implementation of e-learning modules for gatekeepers to prevent suicidality among adolescents.

Simon Hatcher is Professor of Psychiatry at the University of Ottawa, having moved there from Auckland in May 2012. He worked for 18 years in Auckland, New Zealand, as a clinical academic running a Liaison Psychiatry service in a general hospital where he saw many suicidal people in the emergency department and at the Department of Psychological Medicine at the University of Auckland. His main research interests include suicide, self-harm, psychotherapies, psychiatry in the general hospital setting and e-therapies. He provided the clinical input into the John Kirwan Journal program www.depression.org.nz . Currently he is based clinically at the Royal Ottawa Hospital where he is working in an anxiety disorders clinic and providing services in the downtown homeless shelters. Academically, he is based at the University of Ottawa's Institute of Mental Health Research where he is the Cice-Chair of Research in the Department of Psychiatry.

Annemiek Huisman is a post-doctoral researcher at the VU University Amsterdam, the 113Online foundation and the Dutch Health Care Inspectorate. She wrote her Ph.D. thesis on supervision of suicides in mental health care services in the Netherlands (2010) and has continued to study both suicide and the effectiveness of supervision by the Health Care Inspectorate since. Currently, at the VU University, she is developing a Dutch culturally sensitive tool for the assessment of adolescent suicide risk.

Hans M. Koot is Professor of Developmental Psychology and Developmental Psychopathology and Chair of the Department of Developmental Psychology at VU University Faculty of Psychology and Education. He is also Chair of the Mental Health Program at VU University EMGO+ Research Institute.

Karolina Krysinska is a research psychologist working at the Faculty of Psychology and Educational Sciences, KU Leuven, Belgium. Her research interests include risk and protective factors in suicide, suicide prevention, thanatology, psychology of trauma, and psychology of religion. She is an author and co-author of book chapters and peer-reviewed articles on different aspects of suicide, trauma, and bereavement.

Réal Labelle is Professor in the Department of Psychology of the Université du Québec à Montréal (UQAM) and Associate Professor in the Department of Psychiatry of the Université de Montréal (UdeM). He is a researcher at the Centre for Research and Intervention on Suicide and Euthanasia at UQAM and at the Centre de recherche Fernand-Seguin of the UdeM. His university teaching focuses on clinical psychology, particularly cognitive-behavioural approaches. Also, he has been trained in cognitive therapy (CBT) at Beck Institute for Cognitive Therapy and Research in the United States.

Jan. K. Mokkenstorm is the founder, director and a board member of the 113Online Foundation. He specializes in the assessment and (psycho-therapeutic) treatment of suicidal individuals and in the development of e-mental health interventions. His interest in suicidology and research developed in the course of his career as a clinician and administrator of the Department of Acute Psychiatry of GGZ in Geest, a large mental health institute in Amsterdam. He still enjoys working in clinical practice (online and offline) and supervising residents in specialist training. His professional aim is to prevent suicide, to improve access and effectiveness and quality of mental health care, and to develop new innovative practices.

Gillian Murphy has worked in the field of crisis intervention for over 15 years and is Director of Standards, Training and Practices for the National Suicide Prevention Lifeline (Lifeline), a national network of over 160 crisis centers in the United States. In this role, Murphy oversees all aspects of training development with a focus on identifying evidence-based practice and program evaluations that can support the maintenance of recommended practice standards for crisis hotlines. Murphy also oversees the Lifeline's online service delivery through the development of chat- and text-based programs that can provide crisis intervention services to those at risk of suicide. Murphy has extensive experience in community-based crisis intervention and has a background in the management of a primary New York City-based mobile crisis team. She received her Ph.D. in clinical social work from Columbia University.

Xavier Pommereau is a psychiatrist and Director of the Pôle aquitain de l'adolescent at the Centre Abadie of the University Hospital of Bordeaux (CHU) in Bordeaux, France. He has specialized in the treatment of troubled adolescents and suicide prevention. His treatment centre is world renowned for its innovative practices in suicide prevention and the use of new technologies as an adjunct to treatment.

J. H. Smit is the chair for Methodology of Longitudinal Psychiatric Research and Managing Director of Research of the Department of Psychiatry at VU University Medical Centre Amsterdam and Director of the knowledge centre Cohort Research at the VU University Medical Centre. He was originally trained as a Survey Methodologist. He has (co) authored more than 180 peer reviewed international articles.

Bregje A. J. van Spijker is a postdoctoral researcher for the NHMRC Centre for Research Excellence in Suicide Prevention at the Black Dog Institute, Sydney, Australia. She studied the effectiveness of a web-based self-help program aimed at reducing suicidal thoughts in the Netherlands for her Ph.D. and is currently further developing and testing this program in the Australian context.

Christine Thoër is Associate Professor in the Department of Social and Public Communication at the Université du Québec à Montréal and a researcher at the Center on Health Communication (ComSanté). She co-directs the Internet and Health axis of the Quebec Population Health Research Network. Her research focuses on Internet use, especially social networking websites, and their impact on relations between actors and population health.

Carmen E. Vos was a Ph.D. candidate in the Departments of Clinical and Developmental Psychology at VU University Faculty of Psychology and Education, and EMGO+ Institute for Health and Care Research. Her doctoral dissertation is on the development of a self-report instrument for suicidality among adolescents (12–20 years).

David N. Weisstub, a graduate of the Yale Law School, was Professor of Law for over two decades at Osgoode Hall Law School of York University in Toronto. An international consultant on Mental Health Legislation and Forensic reforms, he was invited to become the Philip Pinel Professor of Legal Psychiatry and Bio-medical Ethics at the Université de Montreal in 1993. Editor for 30 years of the *International Journal of Law and Psychiatry*, he has served on numerous editorial boards in the areas of jurisprudence, political theory, bioethics, information technology, and criminology. Currently he is Editor-in-Chief of the *International Library on Ethics Law and the New Medicine* series, published by Springer. Weisstub is legal advisor to both the forensic and torture sections of the World Psychiatric Association. He is a member of the advisory committee to the Federal Minister of Justice of Canada. Honorary life president of the IALMH (International Academy of Law and Mental Health), he is also chairman of its Human Rights Committee. Created a Chevalier in the Legion D'honneur by the Government of France, he also received a knighthood from the Queen of Holland in the order of the Dutch Lion. David has been Chairman of a number of Government inquiries and commissions, including the inquiry in Mental Competency and research ethics with vulnerable populations for the Government of Ontario. He is the author and editor of numerous publications in the field of jurisprudence and mental health law.

1

Suicide Prevention and New Technologies: Towards Evidence Based Practice

Brian L. Mishara and Louis-Philippe Côté

Throughout most of human history people with personal problems would need to seek out another person to obtain help or emotional support. The alternative was to deal with the problem oneself, pray for divine intervention or have some solace from religious beliefs. In more recent times, for those few with the ability and culture to do so, one could also seek information, guidance or support from printed books. The second half of the 20th century was a period when the use of face-to-face professional help expanded throughout the world. During this same period, books became a source of a "do-it-yourself" psychological treatment, with an exponential growth in self-help books for almost any human affliction. In the mid-20th century, a new technology, the telephone, expanded the options for help seeking. Telephone support for suicidal people expanded rapidly since the start of the Samaritan movement in the United Kingdom, founded by Reverend Chad Varah in 1953 (Mishara, 2012). Today, telephone helplines provide crisis intervention, emotional support and suicide prevention services throughout the world. For examples, Befrienders Worldwide has affiliate helplines in more than 40 countries that provide telephone help based upon the Samaritan approach.

Toward the end of the 20th century we witnessed a radical change in help-seeking behaviours, more prominently in developed countries, but rapidly expanding almost everywhere. Today the primary source of information and help for young people considering suicide is the Internet, and the Internet is becoming the principal source of information for all age groups. Furthermore, a large proportion of help seekers on the Internet are looking for information for someone else

(54 per cent according to a US survey of Internet users (PIP, 2000)). The Internet has also become a major means of communications among friends and is increasingly used by people in distress to try to obtain help. The first large-scale Internet-based suicide prevention service was probably begun in July 1994, when the Samaritans of the UK and Republic of Ireland started to respond to e-mails from all over the world from people seeking emotional support (Armson, 1997). Within a few years they were receiving over 500 messages a day, and over 50 per cent of the e-mails expressed feelings of despair and suicide. These messages are automatically sent to over 150 branches and are answered by volunteers who work on the telephone and have received special training on how to reply to e-mail messages.

There is a substantial gap between the exponential growth in use of the Internet to seek help and the slow, sometimes reluctant involvement of professionals and volunteer help givers in providing help over the Internet. This chapter presents an overview of our current understanding of the various current uses of new technologies in suicide prevention, with an emphasis on Internet services. Theories and research on new technologies are still in an embryonic stage, where most of the important issues are just beginning to be explored. Nevertheless, we now have some theoretical perspectives and empirical data to help orient practices.

We live in an age when the emphasis is on *what* to do, with little concern for the theoretical underpinnings of our behaviours. Mishara and colleagues (2007a) reported that when they asked telephone helpline directors to explain what helpers were taught to do over the phones, they could provide detailed descriptions. However, when asked *why* they used those particular intervention methods, they often had little to say, other than to explain that that is what they were taught to do. There was rarely any theoretical or empirical explanation for their current practices. Now, as empirical studies of telephone help are being conducted, we know better what works and what is less effective, and we have better support for some theories than others (e.g. Mishara et al., 2007a; 2007b). In examining practices using new technologies, we often find that methods of intervention are simply transposed from telephone help or face-to-face psychotherapy, with little or no empirical validation of the effectiveness of using these approaches with new technologies. However, there are now some theories and empirical data about new technologies that can offer guidance. This chapter discusses some general theories and their application.

New technologies also pose new ethical challenges. The specific issue of ethical issues in the control of websites that encourage suicide is the subject of the chapter in this book by Mishara and Weisstub (Chapter 5). However, there are ethical choices involved in the use of all new technologies. Again, these choices are rarely explicitly discussed, despite their important implications. The ethical challenges all tend to centre around the rights and obligations of helpers to engage in various suicide prevention activities, with or without overt requests for help from potential suicide victims. Resolving these ethical issues involves the clarification of moral assumptions about the right for people to choose to kill themselves and the obligations in a just society to protect life and help vulnerable populations (See Mishara & Weisstub, 2005; 2007; 2010, for a detailed discussion of these ethical perspectives and their application in suicide prevention).

Some examples to set the stage

This book presents suicide prevention initiatives using new technologies and their application. However, new technologies are not just used to seek help, and help seekers often do not obtain the help they are looking for. Below are a few examples of the range of situations one often encounters:

1. In September 2012, Tyler Clemente, an undergraduate student at Rutgers University, in New Jersey, jumped from the George Washington Bridge after his roommate filmed him having sexual relations with another man. He posted his suicide plans on Facebook. Just before jumping his last post read "Jumping from GW Bridge. Sorry."
2. On Christmas in 2010, a woman in England who had 1082 friends on Facebook posted this message: "I took my pills, I will be dead soon, so good-bye everyone." Many friends did not believe her; some called her a liar, and no one reported her suicide attempt. She died.
3. The Samaritans of the United Kingdom is one of several suicide prevention helplines that responds to SMS text messages. A not uncommon message these helplines receive reads: "I have had enough. I can't continue living."
4. Every day, discussion groups are visited by numerous people discussing their suicidal intentions. One forum in 2012 included the following exchange:
   - Jacques (16 years old): "Everyone would be better off if I were dead"
   - Sylvie (says she is an attractive 16 year old but is actually a known "predator", a man aged 54 who enters discussions on suicide assuming a false identity to encourage people to kill themselves): "Life sucks – I found a good way to end it. So should you. Follow this link to see how to kill yourself easily, painlessly and you won't mess up. I am going to kill myself too. I know how you feel; there is no way out. I'll do it with you."

The number and variety of examples one could cite are immense. One can only conclude that the extensive use of the Internet by suicidal individuals, the extent of help seeking and content that encourages suicide make it imperative that caregivers embrace new technologies and the Internet and as an important means of suicide prevention.

The variety of Internet users: what they are seeking on the Internet

Mixed Expectations: When a person walks into a therapist's office, almost invariably something is troubling the person, and there is a clear expectation that the therapist will help with the client's problems. Callers to telephone helplines, including those dedicated to suicide prevention, are occasionally prank callers who are just amusing themselves; there is even a small proportion who seek sexual stimulation from talking to a stranger, but the vast majority have some sort of problem for which they seek help. These problems range from feeling lonely to being in an acute suicidal crisis with a suicide attempt in progress. Again, the expectations are usually fairly clear: the caller is seeking help, and the helper, who could be a trained lay volunteer or a paid professional, is there to provide that help. However, contacts over the Internet do not require the identification of clearly defined roles. Internet contacts to organizations offering help constitute a very small portion of the Internet activity by suicidal individuals. Suicidal people most often discuss their problems over the Internet with friends and strangers. They can enter a forum; post photographs, videos and messages about their suicidal thoughts or intentions; chat with strangers and seek information about methods to commit suicide; assess their own suicide risk; or even find a partner with whom to commit suicide. There is no intrinsic screening process to identify who is seeking help, which users of which sites are at significant risk of attempting suicide, and which may be considered at low risk or are using the Internet for frivolous purposes. Still, there are a number of clearly identified "danger" signs and indications of an impending or ongoing suicide attempt. People announce their intentions to kill themselves over the Internet on social media sites, there are even examples of real-time videos showing suicide attempts in progress, some attempters send or post farewell letters before their suicide, and some people actively search for the "best" means of ending their lives. Besides people at risk of suicide, there is Internet contact by people who are concerned about the possible suicide of friends or family members and who seek information about what to do to help the suicidal individual.

One may assume that everyone who uses the Internet to make contact or seek information concerning suicide is a potential client or target for suicide prevention activities, regardless of what they purport to be looking for. Some people use the Internet to glorify, publicize, announce or justify their suicide, some try to communicate to others that it is not their fault that they are committing suicide or even to make others feel guilty. People who are not actively seeking referrals or resources for help may still profit from obtaining information about where help may be obtained. Also, people who are not looking for other solutions may still benefit from unsolicited exposure to other ways of dealing with their problems and offers of help, and potential suicide attempts may be avoided.

Variety of Internet Activities: The range of Internet-based activities is constantly expanding and includes video sharing to ask for help and self-help computer programs online to deal with suicidal ideation (see Chapter 6). Online therapy is expanding, as are commemorative sites for people who died by suicide and suicide "games" where an avatar can commit suicide by a choice of methods, and all those activities are subject to controversy and debate about their benefits and dangers. For example, commemorative sites after a suicide may provide helpful support to people bereaved. However, the same sites may be seen as glorifying the suicide, and this could incite others to end their lives in order to posthumously "benefit" from all the attention they will receive and the contrition by people the potential suicide victim feels have been unkind. A study by Eichenberg (2008) of German Internet message boards found that "suicide forums" vary in the help or harm they may provide, with the majority of users seeking constructive help, and only a small minority seeking information on how to commit suicide or partners with whom to commit suicide.

Research has shown (Mesch, 2008) that the choice of different channels or means of Internet communication varies according to different motivations. Mesch (2006) concluded that participation in chat rooms and forums is often motivated by the need for specific, round-the-clock social support. People who need to expand their social network more often use forums and chat rooms, whereas people who want to increase their sense of belonging with their peer group are more likely to use instant messaging, SMS and social networking sites. The research on Internet friendship formation in adolescence and Internet use has focused on two hypotheses: 1) The Rich-Get-Richer Hypothesis proposes that adolescents who already have strong social skills will benefit from the Internet. Research shows that socially anxious and lonely adolescents turn to the Internet for online communication less often than non-socially anxious and non-lonely adolescents. 2) The Social Compensation Hypothesis postulates that lonely and socially anxious adolescents would prefer online communication to face-to-face communication because it is easier to control. However, research has shown that this often does not lead to them establishing new friendships (Valkenburg & Peter, 2011).

There is also some evidence that youth who engage in self-harm have different online behaviours (Mitchell & Ybarra, 2007). Youths who reported deliberate self-harm in the past six months were more likely than other youths to have a sexual screen name or to talk with someone known only online about sex (35 per cent v. 5 per cent) and to use chat rooms (57 per cent v. 29 per cent). Those who engaged in deliberate self-harm were also more likely to have a close relationship with someone they met online (38 per cent v. 10 per cent), and 76 per cent used instant messaging (Mitchell & Ybarra, 2007). Harris, McLean & Sheffield (2009) found that people at high risk of suicide who used the Internet reported less perceived social support from family and friends compared with other online users. They also found that suicide-related online users were less likely to seek help from friends and were more likely to seek help in Internet forums. Suicidal online users found forums to be generally supportive and useful (Eichenberg, 2008; Kral, 2006). They felt that communications with family, health care professionals and help sites were less satisfactory. It appears that suicide-related online users are willing to interact with others, but they have a strong preference for peer-to-peer communications, anonymity and un-moderated formats. These findings tend to support the Social Compensation Hypothesis to explain Internet use by suicidal individuals. According to this theory, people whose social relations are not satisfactory will compensate by seeking social support on the Internet.

Increasing numbers of people use Internet screening sites to determine if they suffer from depression or are at risk of suicide. Leykin, Munoz and Contreras (2012) assessed the depressive and suicidal status of 24,965 users of a depression screening site and concluded that a large proportion of users (67 per cent) screened positive for current major depression and current suicidality (44 per cent), including 7.7 per cent reporting a suicide attempt in the past two weeks. However, of those who participated in monthly follow-ups who had reported a recent suicide attempt, only 37.2 per cent were in treatment for their problems. This highlights a potential disadvantage to online screening. Internet screening usually leaves it to the user of the site to find help. The encouragement to get help the site provides is usually in the form of a written message to the user of the site. Unlike screening performed face to face, where the person conducting the screening can try to motivate suicidal individuals to seek help, make referrals to local resources and even hospitalize a person who is in danger of committing suicide, Internet sites are rarely able to provide local referrals, and their written encouragement to seek help may not be as effective as the insistence of a mental health professional in their community. In this study, the participants who used the screening site came from 86 different countries, making it difficult to include useful local information about resources.

There has been recent concern about the immense popularity of "Massive Multi-player Online Role Playing Games" (MMORPG). These games, where players use avatars to affront challengers in a virtual world, are often described as being addictive. Research has shown that players with problematic game use have low sociability, feel that they lack social support, and are more likely to have aggressive tendencies (Festl, Scharkow & Quandt, 2013; Sublette & Mullan, 2010). Wenzel and colleagues (2009) found, in a Norwegian study of adults, that more time spent playing these games was associated with greater likelihood that the players would report depression, suicidal thoughts and alcohol or drug abuse. A study by Messias and colleagues (2011) found that teens who said they played five hours or more of video games each day were more likely to be sad, have suicidal ideation and suicidal planning, according to a survey they conducted in 2007. This may be due to the tendency of adolescents with depression to isolate themselves, but perhaps get bored of their isolation and seek a surrogate activity that mimics social behaviour but does not provide the same social supports. One of the implications of these findings is that if one were to look for people at higher risk of suicide among Internet users, one place where you would probably find a larger proportion of suicidal individuals would be on platforms with MMORPGs.

The current situation: dangers and benefits

Potential Dangers: The Internet, besides being a source of help in preventing suicides, is also a source of encouragement to proceed with a suicide attempt and a way of learning how to commit suicide. A study by Gunnell and colleagues (2012) investigated the possible use of Internet by people who died by suicide in England. Their assessment of 759 inquest reports in 2005–2007 found that there was evidence of a direct Internet contribution in nine (1.5 per cent) cases. This is most probably an underestimate since inquests into the cause of death do not systematically investigate the Internet use of suicide victims. Of the nine cases Gunnell and colleagues identified, seven people used the Internet to research the method of suicide they used, and five of them had used "unusual" high lethality methods.

One can argue about whether or not there are more pro-suicide or anti-suicide sites on the Internet and whether or not people frequent more often sites which encourage suicide or sites which offer help and support for suicidal individuals. Perhaps it is more important to pay attention to the fact that, according to the study by Marhan and colleagues (2012), people who are looking for information about suicide have a high likelihood of coming across and visiting a site that contains information describing individual suicides without providing any resources for help. This type of suicide content is considered to potentially increase suicide risk and is counter-indicated by the World Health Organization in their guidelines for media reporting (WHO, 2013).

One of the main concerns for people working in suicide prevention has been the fact that there is no control of what suicidal individuals will come across when they search for information or help over the Internet. For example, when Auxéméry and Fidelle (2010) examined which sites a Google search of "suicide pact" would identify, they found that the top 10 sites were journalistic reports about completed suicide pacts that resulted in deaths. However only two of those sites provided any information about how to get help or whom to contact if the visitor was feeling suicidal. Two-thirds gave specific information about the suicide, half had photographs of the event; both are practices which in other media are associated with increased suicide risk (World Health Organization, 2013). Mandrusiak and colleagues (2006) compared the nature of the warning signs for suicide on a random sample of 50 sites from the first 500 hits in a Google search. There were many differences between the warning signs listed on each site, with almost 50 per cent of the "signs" being unique to each site, although most of the major warning signs listed on suicide prevention organization sites were present. Without any control, each site listed what they felt were warning signs for suicide, with more or less agreement with the research data and the opinion of experts in the field.

The total lack of control of the authenticity and usefulness of information and help available online can lead to concerns that vulnerable individuals, who may be more susceptible to imitation or contagion effects, are likely to come across content which increases rather than decreases their suicide risk. In addition, the anonymity of the Internet allows for so-called "predators" to pretend to offer help, but then encourage people to end their lives. There are also issues concerning the security of information people disclose on the Internet, with increasing numbers of people who publicize their suicidal intentions in public over the Internet being identified and having the potential of being mocked or stigmatized for being or having been suicidal.

Although there are examples of group suicides reported for people who met over the Internet in several countries, including Guam and Norway and Korea, the country which appears to have the most Internet group suicides is Japan (Ozawa-De Silva, 2010). Since Internet suicides were recognized by the Japanese police in 2003, the number of group suicides or "suicide pacts" has increased each year. Until 2008, they almost always used the same method of burning charcoal in a small Japanese stove inside a car or apartment with the windows sealed up with tape. Whenever specific information about how to commit suicide using a specific method is promoted over the Internet as a "desirable" way of killing oneself and detailed information is provided about how to use the method, there is a risk that the method will become increasingly popular. In the beginning of 2008, after information of how to commit suicide using hydrogen sulfide poisoning was circulating on the Internet in Japan, that method became extremely popular, and in 2008 there were 1056 suicides using hydrogen sulfide. This new method has now replaced charcoal burning as the preferred method for Internet group suicides and individual suicides in Japan. This points to the power of the Internet to influence the methods used in suicide attempts, with the potential for more lethal consequences.

A typical scenario for an Internet suicide pact in Japan involves people meeting in an online chat and agreeing to commit suicide together at a specific place and time. The mass media in Japan have been reporting on Internet suicide cases with detailed descriptions and have even pointed out where on the Internet individuals can gather to discuss suicide and plan group suicides. For example, after the first Internet suicide occurred in February 2003, there were 599 articles on Internet group suicides in the five major newspapers in Japan and 156 television programmes about Internet group suicides (Ozawa-De-Silva, 2010). The more the news media reported on suicide pacts where people met over the Internet, the more frequently suicide pacts occurred.

Potential Benefits: The potential benefits of using the Internet to help people who are suicidal are many. First, the simple fact that the Internet is a primary source of information implies that suicide prevention organizations need to have a presence and offer services over the Internet that are compatible with the help-seeking patterns of the population. Even without the involvement of suicide prevention organizations, the social support, information and help that many people obtain over the Internet may be a powerful protective factor for suicidal individuals. Internet users may learn about and subsequently imitate positive role models, persons who have had similar problems but found solutions and reasons to go on living. In this realm of possible anonymity, people who are concerned about the stigma that may be associated with feeling suicidal or talking about suicide may feel more at ease. Furthermore, the Internet provides the potential for identifying high-risk individuals who are seriously considering suicide and then targeting interventions to this population. There is also the potential benefit of cost reduction, since automated programmes providing self-diagnosis and self-help can facilitate maximum use of costly human resources to provide treatment and crisis intervention services to those who are truly in need and those who do not benefit from self-help programmes.

When we examine the current situation, we find a great number of specific initiatives with little integration and coordination. Both Google and Yahoo will show links to telephone helplines in the United-States when someone searches for "suicide methods" in English (see Chapter 9 by Murphy). In some other countries, for example in Belgium, they have established agreements with organizations who are able to provide help. Facebook has a rather complicated mechanism to "report story or spam" through which, after going through several pages ("if story is found abusive, file a report," then "violence or harmful behaviour," then a menu which includes "self-harm" and then "suicidal content"), one will eventually be able to click on "report suicidal content page". Then, in the United States, the phone number and contact information for the National Suicide Prevention Lifeline (NSPL) will be sent to the person, and the NSPL will be informed and, depending upon their assessment of the suicide risk in the situation, may initiate contact with the suicidal individual.

In terms of controlling "dangerous" sites, Australia currently has a national law which forbids Internet Services Providers (ISPs) to provide access to sites that encourage suicide or provide information on means for killing oneself. Chapter 5, by Mishara and Weisstub, discusses the ethical, legal and practical concerns on banning Internet sites or blocking access, as well as the potential advantages and disadvantages of such actions.

There is a full range of services offered in different countries using the Internet and portable telephone technologies, including cognitive behavioural therapy provided online, chats with trained helpers, monitored forums for suicidal individuals, help offered in reply to e-mails, automated self-help programmes for suicidal preoccupations and automated programmes for smartphones that can check on the well-being of suicidal individuals, including people who have attempted suicide who may be at risk of a repeated attempt, with automated calls for help to social supports and professionals in a crisis situation.

Need for evaluation

Despite the proliferation of Internet activities, few existing practices are based on empirical data proving their efficacy. Most involve transforming practices in face-to-face and telephone help to the media of the Internet. Still, several training modules explaining how to apply methods used in other practices to the Internet appear to have some erroneous assumptions. Our perusal of various training manuals indicates that they often have a discussion of the fact that since information such as tone of voice and visual expressions are not available over the Internet, it is more difficult to communicate empathy and understanding. However, the issue of the extent of self-disclosure over the Internet in comparison with face-to-face communication is complex. The meta-analysis by Nguyen, Bin and Campbell (2012) examined 15 empirical studies that made 24 comparisons between online and offline self-disclosure. They found that equal numbers of studies found greater online self-disclosure, greater face-to-face disclosure and no difference between online and offline disclosure. It appears that empathy may in fact be more difficult to communicate online. However, there is a general tendency to idealize the person one is communicating with online, and this tendency may lead to greater self-disclosure even if the helper is not as effective in communicating empathetic understanding. Also, it may be that disclosure over the Internet occurs as a process that is independent of what the helper communicates, as the result of an inherent need to share one's life that is facilitated by the medium of the Internet. For example, there has been a recent growth of "confession" sites where people can anonymously post descriptions of things they did that were not nice and possibly illegal.

Issues and challenges

Peers versus trained helpers and professionals

One of the issues in Internet suicide prevention concerns the relative advantages and disadvantages of online lay mutual help or self-help groups when compared to help from suicide prevention agencies and professional organizations. There is some evidence that online peer communities are perceived as being helpful and have the advantage that adolescents, in particular, feel more comfortable seeking help online for personal issues, including thoughts about suicide (Greidanus & Everall, 2010).

There is a difference between how peers interact with people who are suicidal and in distress in Internet forums and how volunteers in suicide prevention interact, at least according to studies conducted in Israel (Gilat, Tobin & Shahar, 2011). Volunteers tend to use more cognitive change techniques, interpretation and empowerment, which are interpreted as being "cognitive focused therapeutic like" and give more moral support than peers. Generally, peers are perceived as quite helpful to young people in distress. For example, Fukkink (2011) found that on scales of 1 to 9 peer volunteers had an overall average score of 7.1 in terms of emotional support strategies provided. However, peers less often tended to offer solutions or encouraged the person to think about solutions for solving the problem.

In Israel, helpers tended to respond differently to messages in an online forum from suicidal individuals, depending upon the nature of the situation. For example, when a suicide attempt appeared to be imminent, 71 per cent tried to discourage them from proceeding with the suicide attempt by arguing why they should not do so. However, when suicidal people talked about loneliness, they were often offered group support.

Not all results are positive. For example, Barak and Dolev-Cohen (2006) found that participation in a forum did not significantly reduce distress in suicidal adolescents. Still, those who posted more messages and received more replies had lower levels of distress in the following months. It is important to conduct studies of Internet help provided by both peers and trained helpers in different cultural contexts before generalizing results from one society to another. To date, we know very little about the relative effectiveness of different forms of online support in actually presenting suicide.

Computer programs replacing and complementing human therapists and helpers

There has been much discussion of whether or not one day a computer can replace a psychotherapist, and there are many psychotherapy programs which have been tested, with varying degrees of success. The Holy Grail of using a computer to replace a human is the Turing test proposed by Turing (1950) to determine whether or not machines can think. The idea is not to answer that philosophical question specifically, but rather to ascertain if digital computers can do well in imitating humans by having someone question another person and a machine in order to determine which is the machine and which is the human being. Although it does not appear that we now have a computer that is capable of passing the Turing test to the satisfaction of the most diligent researchers, psychotherapy programs are being used increasingly with suicidal individuals, and their potential in preventing suicides needs to be evaluated.

Recent research has focused on the potential of using machine-learning algorithms (MLA) to determine if someone is at risk of committing suicide or not. Computer applications have been used to compare simulated and actual notes left by people who completed suicide. For example, Pestian and colleagues (2008) used an algorithm that was accurate 71 per cent of the time, compared to mental health professionals who were accurate 78 per cent of the time, but this difference was not statistically significant. Another study (Pestian et al., 2010) found that mental health professionals in training were accurate 49 per cent of the time in identifying the actual suicide notes, compared to mental health professionals 63 per cent, but the computer algorithm was accurate 78 per cent of the time. It is one thing to retrospectively compare a suicide note to a "mock" note created for the purpose of conducting an experiment. However, the comparison may not be realistic since people who do not attempt suicide generally do not leave fake suicide notes.

There is a growing number of studies that attempt to analyze levels of distress and other affective states in written texts (Lehrman et al., 2012). For example, Haerian and colleagues (2012) used natural language processing (NLP) to analyze electronic health records in order to see if they could identify patients with suicidal thoughts or behaviours, and they compared this to diagnoses using the ECD-9 E-code algorithm. Although these efforts are at an embryonic stage, it is possible that in the future computers will be able to scan Internet communications in various formats and identify people's levels of distress and risk of attempting suicide, or analyze records, tests or interview recordings to identify suicide risk.

Some researchers suggest that people who attempt suicide are more comfortable participating in a computer interview to assess suicide risk than a face-to-face evaluation by a physician. Petrie & Abell (1994) asked 150 hospitalized patients who had attempted suicide if they would prefer a computer interview or an interview with a doctor. 52 per cent preferred the computer compared to 17.4 per cent the doctor, and 30 per cent had no preference. Patients with higher levels of suicidal ideation and hopelessness, and lower levels of self-esteem were more likely to prefer the computer.

There is evidence that automated Internet treatment for depression using a cognitive behavioural therapy approach may be associated with decreases in suicidal ideation and depression (Watts et al., 2012). Chapter 6 of this book by Ghoncheh and colleagues presents an automated programme to decrease suicidal thinking.

Research and theories of how communication over the Internet is different

The psychology of writing as therapy

Most current Internet communications use writing rather than verbal communications. Research by psychologists who have studied the differences between written and verbal communication methods may be relevant to understanding how written communications over the Internet may be best used in suicide prevention. When people write, they tend to express things that might not be expressed at all in other modes of communication (Barak, 2007; Pennebaker et al., 2003; Barak and Miron, 2005). These differences have been attributed to the experience of aloneness in writing, a sense of complete privacy (Ben-Ze'ev, 2003; Viseu et al., 2004) that produces a "feeling of self-talk" that cannot occur when another person is present. Furthermore, writing over the Internet allows for messages to be easily saved, retrieved, copied, forwarded, encrypted and backed-up, and then sent only when the writer is ready to send the message. This flexibility in when to send a message or reply to a written message, called "elasticity of synchronicity" (Newhagen and Rafaeli, 1996) or "temporal fluidity" (Suler, 2004), allows for better control by the person who is writing. Writers can take the time they want to reflect upon what they are writing before sending each written communication. When communicating in-person face to face, reactions tend to be immediate, and the time to reflect before responding is limited by the social pressure to reply immediately.

There have been a number of studies of the use of writing as a psychotherapy tool. Smyth (1998) conducted a meta-analysis of 13 studies of writing therapies and found a general significant positive effect on psychological well-being and general functioning. Positive results were more likely to occur with men, people with medical problems, difficulties identifying feelings and people who tend to see things as either black or white, and people with more severe clinical symptoms (Baikie & Wilhem, 2005). There are indications that writing about problems may result in some short-term distress, but the longer-term effects tend to be beneficial. According to Pennebaker (2004), the potential benefits of writing about one's problems in a therapeutic context are associated with a complex combination of immediate cognitive and/or emotional changes, longer-term cognitive and/or emotional changes, social processes and biological effects. The most helpful writings about one's problems are when the writer includes both thoughts and feelings ("cognitions and emotions") (Pennebaker & Beall, 1986; Smyth & Pennebaker, 1999).

Self-disclosure: Nguyen, Bin and Campbell (2012) conducted a systematic review of self-disclosure online and off-line. There are several dimensions to self-disclosure that have been studied. The frequency of self-disclosure refers to the amount of information revealed. There is also the range or diversity of self-disclosure, which is referred to as "disclosure breadth". Also, one can assess the intimacy of personal information divulged, called the "depth" of self-disclosure. This review found that, although several studies found greater online disclosure using these different dimensions, it was not always the case. Disclosure is content specific. When there are few individuating cues, exaggerated intimacy is more likely. Also, when social norms are not present, individuals are more likely to be disinhibited and will disclose more freely. Overall, remaining invisible to others on the Internet and not being able to see others tends to make one more susceptible to group norms and more likely to share (disclose) intimate details of one's life (Walther, 2011). Researchers have found that disclosure and personal questions constitute greater proportions of utterances in online discussions among strangers than they do in comparable face-to-face discussions (Joinson, 2001; Tidwell & Walther, 2002).

This increased self-disclosure can be a double-edged sword in terms of suicide prevention. It makes it easier for helpers to learn about the person and the risk of suicide. On the other hand, too much self-disclosure to strangers over the Internet can lead to people learning things one may not want to be shared for everyone to see. Also, self-disclosure on the Internet by vulnerable people may sometimes make people more susceptible to persons who try to encourage others to commit suicide.

There is also research on self-presentation online and how people modify how they present themselves as a function of their expectations of what the other people would think or are looking for, as well as what they themselves might want to be or how they would like to see themselves. Gonzalez and Hancock (2008) suggest that not only these differences in individuals' construction of stories about themselves online influence how others see them, but they also can transform the individuals' self-perception. They call this phenomenon "identity shift". This would suggest that if people involved in suicide prevention are able to entice suicidal individuals to present themselves as non-suicidal, at least in theory (but perhaps in practice as well), they may begin to see themselves as non-suicidal.

Response delays, the possibility to edit before sending and the ability to easily end an Internet contact: In computer-mediated communication, there are usually response delays that are much greater than in verbal communications. We know little about the implications of these delays on how to be most helpful over the Internet. There are many research questions which need to be answered. In face-to-face therapy one cannot suddenly "turn-off" and terminate the session at will. There is great social pressure to stay in the room and continue the conversation. However, over the Internet one can simply stop the conversation at any time without consequence. This provides a great level of control for the person seeking help and can be a great source of stress for helpers. We know little about the best practices to keep Internet conversations going and very little about the impact of Internet users having greater control on the effectiveness of different forms and methods of providing help over the Internet.

Another characteristic of Internet communications is the ability to edit messages (deletions, backspaces and insertions) before sending them. The amount of editing people use varies according to different characteristics of the users and their perceptions of the person(s) with whom they are interacting. For example, there is more editing when the person with whom one is communicating is perceived as more desirable (Walther, 2007). Also, people who self-reported higher levels of mindfulness during message production spent more time editing their messages, and persons who were lower in mindfulness spent more time choosing what to write before typing.

How to be helpful over the Internet and differences with telephone help

Studies in Israel found that suicide threats were rare in online chats (only 1 in the 373 chats studied) and uncommon in telephone interventions (1.5 per cent, 64 calls out of 4426), but much more common in forums (15.3 per cent, 146 suicidal messages out of 954 messages). However, one can question those results. Many suicide helplines in North America have suicidal ideation in 50 per cent of calls (Mishara et al., 2007b) and most helplines have a much higher percentage of suicidal calls than the 15 per cent they found in online forums in Israel. This may reflect differences in their approaches to intervention: most North-American helplines have a policy of always asking direct questions about suicidal ideation. If questions about suicide are always asked, it is likely that more suicide intentions will be revealed.

Recent research on which methods of intervention are most effective in telephone help with people in a suicidal crisis (Mishara et al., 2007a; 2007b) have found that a more directive problem-solving approach is associated with positive changes and a non-directive Rogerian approach was not necessarily helpful in a suicidal crisis. One of the findings in their study, which is often ignored, was that the benefits of the more directive, collaborative problem-solving approach were found to only hold in situations where a good contact with the client was made by an empathetic and respectful helper in the first three minutes of the call. Generally, this good contact involving empathy and respect is established using classical non-directive Rogerian techniques. One can ask if these results can be transposed to online help, particularly one-to-one help provided in Internet chat services.

There is increasing recognition that suicide prevention services may need to be adapted according to the sex of the client. Telephone help services tend to have more female callers than males (sometimes as many as two women for each man), but online chats have an even higher proportion of female participants, between 72 per cent and 89 per cent (Drexler, 2012; Meunier, 2011; Mokkenstorm, 2012; Kids Helpline, 2012; Tanaka, 2011). Users of Internet services to obtain help tend to have more distress than telephone callers, have more severe problems and are often already involved with some form of mental health services.

There have been several evaluations of chat services. However, these evaluations rarely focus specifically on suicidal callers nor have used outcome variables measuring suicidal ideation or attempts. A study of the Australian Kids Helpline (Chardon, Bagraith & King, 2011) found that their chats spent most of the time exploring the problem but rarely did much in the way of trying to find solutions. Furthermore, in only 53 per cent of the cases they followed the model they were supposed to use according to their training. It may simply be that it takes so much time exploring the problems that they never get to begin exploring solutions, as suggested by Bambling and colleagues (2008).

Timm (2011) suggested that when online helpers adopt the communication style of the client (using their type of informal language) and explain why they are asking potentially delicate questions before asking them, the impact is more positive. However, asking a series of questions, for example as part of an inventory to assess suicide risk, tends to have a negative impact. Some specific techniques may be helpful. The technique of "normalization" (Shea, 1999), in which the helper explains that people in that person's particular situation sometimes think of suicide before asking if that person is considering suicide, may elicit more disclosure of suicidal ideation. Another technique is to sandwich a more delicate directive question between two empathetic statements. ("You really have had a horrible shock being dumped like that. Put your pills away and let's talk about what can be done. You seem so frustrated and alone." or "You are very upset about how he reacted. Have you thought of apologizing to him? The situation seems so difficult for you.")

In conclusion

Many years ago the prestigious psychology professor Heinz Werner was conducting a seminar for doctoral students at Clark University, and he said to his students, "In the future, everything that you have learnt in this course will be obsolete." A graduate student asked, "So, why am I spending countless hours learning about all this?" Werner replied, "I hope that what I am teaching becomes obsolete, because that will indicate that people have paid attention to what I have to say and will have learnt from it and have progressed." In the area of suicide prevention and new technologies, most of the potential is yet to be discovered, and we would hope that our current presentation of evidence-based practices will be replaced by more sophisticated and extensive research findings and theories. In the coming years, our relationship to the Internet and computerized devices will change and expand in ways we have not yet conceived. We look forward to these new developments, but hope that the evidence base to identify best practices increases in parallel to the increased development and use of these new services.

References

Armson, S. (1997). Suicide and Cyberspace-Befriending by e-mail. *Crisis, 18*(3), 103–106.

Auxéméry, Y., & Fidelle, G. (2010). Impact d'internet sur la suicidalité. À propos d'une "googling study" sur la retro-information médiatique d'un pacte pacte suicidaire échafaudé sur le web. *Annales Médico-Psychologiques, 168*(7), 502–507.

Baikie, K. A., & Wilhem, K. (2005). Emotional and physical health benefits of expressive writing. *Advances in Psychiatric Treatment, 11*(5), 338–346.

Bambling, M., King, R., Reid, W., & Wegner, K. (2008). Online counselling: The experience of counsellors providing synchronous single-session counselling to young people. *Counselling and Psychotherapy Research, 8*(2), 110–116.

Barak, A. (2007). Phantom emotions: Psychological determinants of emotional experiences on the Internet. In A. Joinson, K. Y. A. McKenna, T. Postmes, & U. D. Reips (eds), *Oxford handbook of Internet psychology* (pp. 303–329). Oxford, UK: Oxford University Press.

Barak, A., & Dolev-Cohen, M. (2006). Does activity level in online support groups for distressed adolescents determine emotional relief? *Counselling and Psychotherapy Research, 6*(3), 186–190.

Barak, A., & Miron, O. (2005). Writing characteristics of suicidal people on the Internet: A psychological investigation of emerging social environments. *Suicide and Life-Threatening Behavior, 35*(5), 507–524.

Ben-Ze'ev, A. (2003). Privacy, emotional closeness, and openness in cyberspace. *Computers in Human Behavior, 19*(4), 451–467.

Chardon, L., Bagraith, K. S., & King, R. J. (2011). Counseling activity in single-session online counseling with adolescents: An adherence study. *Psychotherapy Research, 21*(5), 583–592.

Drexler, M. (2012, May). CrisisChat.org : Online emotional support : A program of CONTACT USA. Paper presented at the Centre for Research and Intervention on Suicide and Euthanasia Ninth Summer Institute, Montreal, QC. Retrieved 6 August 2012, from http://www.crise.ca/pdf/CRISE-Summer-Institute-2012-Drexler.pdf

Eichenberg, C. (2008). Internet message boards for suicidal people: A typology of users. *CyberPsychology and Behavior, 11*(1), 107–113.

Festl, R., Scharkow, M., & Quandt, T. (2013). Problematic computer game use among adolescents, younger and older adults. *Addiction, 108*(3), 592–599.

Fukkink, R. (2011). Peer counseling in an online chat service: A content analysis of social support. *Cyberpsychology, Behaviour and Social Networking, 14*(4), 247–251.

Gilat, I., Tobin, Y., & Shahar, G. (2011). Offering support to suicidal individuals in an online support group. *Archives of Suicide Research, 15*(3), 195–206.

Gonzales, A. L., & Hancock, J. T. (2008). Identity shift in computer-mediated environments. *Media Psychology, 11*(2), 167–185.

Greidanus, E., & Everall, R. D. (2010). Helper therapy in an online suicide prevention community. *British Journal of Guidance & Counselling, 38*(2), 191–204.

Gunnell, D., Bennewith, O., Kappur, N., Simkin, S., Cooper, J., & Hawton, K. (2012). The use of the internet by people who die by suicide in England: A cross sectional study. *Journal of Affective Disorders, 141*, 480–483.

Haerian, K., Salmasian, H., & Friedman, C. (2012). Methods for Identifying Suicide and Suicidal Ideation in EHRs. Paper presented at the AMIA Annual Symposium Proceedings, 1244–1253.

Harris, K. M., McLean, J. P., & Sheffield, J. (2009). Examining suicide-risk individuals who go online for suicide-related purposes. *Archives of Suicide Research, 14*(3), 206–221.

Joinson, A. N. (2001). Self-disclosure in computer-mediated communication: The role of self-awareness and visual anonymity. *European Journal of Social Psychology, 31*(2), 177–192.

Kids Helpline. (2012). Overview 2011. Brisbane: Kids Helpline. Retrieved 6 August 2012 from http://www.kidshelp.com.au/upload/22918.pdf

Kral, G. (2006). Online communities for mutual help: Fears, fiction, and facts. In M. Murero, & R. E. Rice (eds), *The Internet and health care: Theory, research, and practice* (pp. 215–232). Mahwah, NJ: Lawrence Erlbaum Associates.

Lehrman, M. T., Alm, C. O., & Proano, R. A. (2012). *Detecting distressed and non-distressed affect states in short forum texts.* Paper presented at the Proceedings of the Second Workshop on Language in Social Media.

Leykin, Y., Munoz, R. F., & Contreras, O. (2012). Are consumers of internet health information "cyberchondriacs"? Characteristics of 24,965 users of a depression screening site. *Depression and Anxiety, 29,* 71–77.

Mandrusiak, M., Rudd, M. D., Joiner, T. E., Berman, A. L., Van Orden, K. A., & Witte, T. (2006). Warning signs for suicide on the Internet: A descriptive study. *Suicide and Life-Threatening Behavior, 36*(3), 263–271.

Marhan, A. M., Săucan, D., Popa, C., & Danciu, B. (2012). Searching Internet: A report on accessibility, nature, and quality of suicide-related information. *Procedia – Social and Behavioral Sciences, 33,* 373–377.

Mesch, G. (2006). Online communities. In R. Cnaan, & C. Milofsky (eds), *Handbook of Community and Community Organization.* New York: Springer

—— (2008). Internet Affordances and Teens' Social Communication: From Diversification to Bonding. In R. Zheng, J. Burrow-Sanchez, & C. Drew (eds), *Adolescent online social communication and behavior: Relationship formation on the internet* (pp. 14–28). Hershey, PA: Information Science Reference.

Messias, E., Castro, J., Saini, A., Usman, M., & Peeples, D. (2011). Sadness, suicide, and their association with video game and internet overuse among teens: results from the Youth Risk Behavior Survey 2007 and 2009. *Suicide and Life-Threatening Behavior, 41*(3), 307–315.

Meunier, P. (2011). www.chat-accueil.org: Un outil jeune pour un public jeune [A young tool for a young public]. Brussels: Télé-Accueil Bruxelles. Retrieved 6 August 2012, from http://www.tele-accueil- bruxelles.be/files/pdf/Chat_Accueil_outil_pr_public_jeune.pdf

Mishara, B. L. (2012). How to help suicidal persons over the telephone and Internet. In D. Lester, & J. R. Rogers (eds), *Crisis intervention and counseling by telephone and the internet* (3rd ed.) (pp. 74–84). Springfield, IL: Charles C. Thomas.

Mishara, B. L. Chagnon, F., Daigle, M., Balan, B., Raymond, S., Marcoux, I., Bardon, C., Campbell, J. K., & Berman, A. (2007a). Comparing models of helper behavior to actual practice in telephone crisis intervention: A silent monitoring study of calls to the U.S. 1–800-SUICIDE Network. *Suicide and Life-Threatening Behavior, 37*(3), 293–309.

—— (2007b). Which helper behaviors and intervention styles are related to better short-term outcomes in telephone crisis intervention? Results from a silent monitoring study of calls to the U.S. 1–800-SUICIDE Network. *Suicide and Life-Threatening Behavior, 37*(3), 310–323.

Mishara, B. L., & Weisstub, D. N.(2005). Ethical issues in suicide research. *International Journal of Law and Psychiatry, 28*, 23–41.

—— (2007). Ethical, legal, and practical issues in the control and regulation of suicide promotion and assistance over the Internet. *Suicide and Life-Threatening Behavior, 37*(1), 58–65.

—— (2010). Resolving ethical dilemmas in suicide prevention: The case of telephone helpline rescue policies. *Suicide and Life-Threatening Behavior, 40*(2), 159–169.

Mitchell, K. J., & Ybarra, M. L. (2007). Online behavior of youth who engage in self-harm provides clues for preventive intervention. *Preventive Medicine, 45*, 392–396.

Mokkenstorm, J. (2012, May). 113ONLINE: Education, help and intervention with people on the Internet. Paper presented at the Centre for Research and Intervention on Suicide and Euthanasia Ninth Summer Institute, Montreal, QC. Retrieved 6 August 2012, from http://www.crise.ca/pdf/CRISE-Summer-Institute-2012-Mokkenstorm.pdf

Newhagen, J. E. & Rafaeli, S. (1996).Why communication researchers should study the Internet: A dialogue. *Journal of Computer-Mediated Communication* 1(4), Retrieved 12 March 2012 from http://jcmc.indiana.edu/vol1/issue4/rafaeli.html

Nguyen, M., Bin, Y. S., & Campbell, A. (2012). Comparing online and offline self-disclosure: A systematic review. *Cyberpsychology, Behavior, and Social Networking, 15*(2), 103–111.

Ozawa-De Silva, C. (2010). Shared death: self, sociality and internet group suicide in Japan. *Transcultural Psychiatry, 47*(3), 392–418.

Pennebaker, J. W. (2004). Theories, therapies, and taxpayers: On the complexities of the expressive writing paradigm. *Clinical Psychology: Science and Practice, 11*, 138–142.

Pennebaker, J. W., & Beall, S. K. (1986). Confronting a traumatic event: Toward an understanding of inhibition and disease. *Journal of Abnormal Psychology, 95*, 274–281.

Pennebaker, J. W., Mehl, M. R., & Niederhoffer, K. G. (2003). Psychological aspects of natural language use: Our words, our selves. *Annual Review of Psychology, 54*, 547–577.

Pestian, J. P., Matykiewicz, P., & Grupp-Phelan, J. (2008). *Using natural language processing to classify suicide notes.* Paper presented at the Proceedings of the Workshop on Current Trends in Biomedical Natural Language Processing.

Pestian, J., Nasrallah, H., Matykiewicz, P., Bennett, A., & Leenaars, A.(2010). Suicide note classification using natural language processing: A content analysis. *Biomedical Informatics Insights, 3*, 19.

Petrie, K., & Abell, W. (1994). Responses of parasuicides to a computerized interview. *Computers in Human Behavior, 10*(4), 415–418.

PIP (2000). Pew Internet and American life project: Online life report. Retrieved 15 June 2013, from http://www.pewinternet.org/reports/pdfs/PIP_Health_Report.pdf

Shea, S. C. (1999). *The practical art of suicide assessment: A guide for mental health professionals and substance abuse counsellors.* New York: John Wiley & Sons.

Smyth, J. M. (1998). Written emotional expression: Effect sizes, outcome types, and moderating variables. *Journal of Consulting and Clinical Psychology, 66,* 174–184.

Smyth, J. M. & Pennebaker, J. W. (1999) Sharing one's story: translating emotional experiences into words as a coping tool. In C. R. Snyder (ed.), *Coping: The psychology of what works,* (pp. 70–89). New York: Oxford University Press.

Sublette, V.A., & Mullan, B. (2012). Consequences of play : A systematic review of the effects of online gaming. *International Journal of Mental Health and Addiction, 10*(1), 3–23.

Suler, J. (2004). The psychology of text relationships. In R. Kraus, J. Zack, & G. Stricker (eds), *Online counseling: A handbook for mental health professionals* (pp. 19–50). San Diego, CA: Academic Press Elsevier. Retrieved 3 March 2012, from http://users.rider.edu/~suler/psycyber/psytextrel.html

Tanaka, J. (2011, October). YouthInBC.com: What the past seven years have taught us (and what we still have to learn). Paper presented at the 2011 Canadian Association of Suicide Prevention National Conference, Vancouver, BC.

Tidwell, L. C., & Walther, J. B. (2002). Computer-mediated communication effects on disclosure, impressions, and interpersonal evaluations: Getting to know one another a bit at a time. *Human Communication Research, 28*(3), 317–348.

Timm, M. (2011). Crisis counselling online: Building rapport with suicidal youth. (Master of Arts – MA), University of British Columbia, Vancouver. Retrieved from Williams, R., Bambling, M., King, R., & Abbott, Q. (2009). In-session process in online counselling with young people: An exploratory approach. *Counselling and Psychotherapy Research, 9*(2), 93–100.

Turing, A. M. (1950). Computing machinery and intelligence. *Mind, 59*(236), 433–460.

Valkenburg, P. M., & Peter, J. (2011). Online communication among adolescents: An integrated model of its attraction, opportunities, and risks. *The Journal of Adolescent Health: Official publication of the Society for Adolescent Medicine, 48*(2), 121–127.

Viseu, A., Clement, A., & Aspinall, J. (2004). Situating privacy online: Complex perceptions and everyday practices. *Information, Communication & Society, 7*(1), 92–114.

Walther, J. B. (1994) [2007]). Selective self-presentation in computer-mediated communication: Hyperpersonal dimensions of technology, language, and cognition. *Computers in Human Behavior, 23*(5), 2538–2557.

—— (2011). Theories of computer-mediated communications and interpersonal relations. In M. L. Knapp, & J. A. Daly (eds), T*he Handbook of Interpersonal Communication* (4th ed.) (pp. 443–479). Thousand Oaks, CA: Sage.

Watts, S., Newby, J. M., Mewton, L., & Andrews, G. (2012). A clinical audit of changes in suicide ideas with internet treatment for depression. *British Medical Journal Open, 2*(5), 2: e001558.

Wenzel, H., Bakken, I., Johansson, A., Götestam, K., & Øren, A. (2009). Excessive computer game playing among Norwegian adults: Self-reported consequences of playing and association with mental health problems. *Psychological Reports,* *105*(3F), 1237–1247.

World Health Organization (2013). *Preventing suicide: A resource for media professionals.* http://www.who.int/mental_health/prevention/suicide/resource_media.pdf Retrieved on 24 April 2013.

2

Expressing, Communicating and Discussing Suicide: Nature, Effects and Methods of Interacting through Online Discussion Platforms

Christine Thoër

In many countries, the Internet is a source frequently used to look up health information (Fox & Duggan, 2013; McDaid &Park, 2010). Several surveys conducted in the United States have focused on the increasingly important role that social media plays in providing access to health information (Health Research Institute, 2012; The Change Foundation, 2011a; Chou et al., 2009; Fox & Jones, 2009). Social media platforms are especially popular among teens and young adults researching sensitive topics such as sexuality, mental health, drug use including recreational use of prescription medication, and self-harm (Buhi et al., 2009; Gray et al., 2005; Gray & Klein, 2006; Harvey et al., 2007; Tackett-Gibson, 2007, 2008; Thoër & Aumond, 2010; Aubé & Thoër, 2009; Whitlock, Powers & Eckenrode, 2006). On these platforms, individuals are exposed to information from numerous sources, including governments, health institutions, health professionals, private health service providers and, most importantly, peers and family members (Romeyer, 2008).

Exposure to stories about suicide typically occurs through traditional media (64 per cent) and friends and relatives (55 per cent). Informational websites (44 per cent), social networking sites (24 per cent) and forums, chat rooms and online message boards (15 per cent) are also widely consulted information sources for people experiencing mental health problems and suicidal ideation; these people are frequent users of blogs and other online discussion forums between peers (Dunlop, More & Romer, 2011; Niezen, 2013). Studies have shown a correlation between addiction to the Internet, which has sometimes been called, "pathological use of the Internet" and self-harm and suicidal ideation in young people (Durkee et al., 2011). It is therefore especially important to get a clearer picture of what happens in online discussions about suicide. In this chapter, which is based on a review of the scientific literature, we will first present the particularities of social media with regards to information flow. Then, we will explore the types of suicide information being disseminated on these platforms, especially forums, which are the most documented type of online discussion, and the effects of using these platforms. We will also discuss users' methods of interacting, which are not well documented for forums and chat rooms; this will lead us to expand our review of the literature to include works about recreational use of medication. We will conclude by highlighting the limitations of works dealing with online discussions about suicide, identifying areas for future research.

New interfaces for information about suicide

Social media has many specific characteristics that differentiate it from traditional media: methods of disseminating health information, the type of content shared, and even the impact their use has on attitudes and behavioural intentions (Renaud, 2012). One of these first characteristics shared by all information available online is the fact that research is active. As the Internet is accessible at all times and low-cost, users can research suicide whenever they feel that this problem concerns them, either personally or because of a loved one, and they are much more receptive to what they learn.

Furthermore, although social media platforms offer an extensive range of health information, they are first and foremost spaces for dialogue and sharing experiences (Thoër, 2012). This focus on experience encourages appropriation of information, as it relates directly to Internet users' daily worries and is more practical, more accessible (Akrich & Méadel, 2002; 2009) and often illustrated (Morey et al., 2011). The fact that this information is being discussed between peers also contributes to changes in attitudes and behavioural intentions, as pointed out by different surveys on prevention and health promotion (Renaud, 2012). Finally, peers, especially those with some experience, become role models with whom Internet users can identify, and who, according to Bandura's social cognitive theory (1977), could help to spread the practices being discussed. Social media would therefore modify the way in which individuals access information about health, with users now relying less on traditional specialists and established institutions (Eysenbach, 2008). The role played by "lay experts" seems greater when it involves behaviours that call health professionals into question (see Thoër & Aumond, 2011, concerning medicated weight loss).

Another feature of social media, and more specifically forums, is that they benefit from strong search engine placement: items published by Internet users help to renew website content, which is one of the characteristics used by the search engines that index Internet resources. Moreover, on social networking sites such as Facebook, which are very popular with teens and young adults, people have access to a more extensive knowledge network, largely due to updates from loose acquaintances, which increases their exposure to suicide stories presented in different formats (videos, stories, testimonials, etc. ...) (Dunlop, More & Romer, 2011). News websites have also promoted the spread of information about cybersuicides, which are frequently picked up by the online press, ignoring WHO recommendations on how to present suicide in the media in order to reduce contagion effects (Auxéméry & Fidelle, 2010).

The wide variety of suicide information available online

Forums, which are one of the oldest social media platforms dedicated to health, are very heterogeneous spaces, which can be free or moderated, open to the public or requiring prior registration (which seems to be the case for many discussion forums about suicide). They come from a wide range of sources (individuals, user groups, community organizations, health professionals, etc.) and follow different philosophies; as a result, the nature and quality of information provided is rather varied (Herbert, Rioux & Brunet, 2012; Thoër, 2012).

Many authors have attempted to provide an overview of the content available online for suicide, including content circulating on social media platforms. For most of these studies, the corpus being analyzed was created by entering a number of keywords relating to suicide into major search engines, then limiting the results to specific geographic zones: China (Cheng et al., 2011), Great Britain (Biddle et al., 2008), United States (Recupero, Harms & Noble 2008), and Turkey (Sakarya, Güneş & Sakarya, 2013). The first resources that appeared for each of the keywords were subject to content analysis intended to determine if the information presented effectively deals with suicide, is "pro-suicide," neutral, or favourable to suicide prevention. Results show that between 5 per cent and 40 per cent of the sites analyzed glorify suicide, with a sizable portion of their content being information on how to end one's life. Furthermore, while some sites presented methods for ending one's life in a very factual manner, without encouraging suicide (Biddle et al., 2008), these resources could still help to complete the transition from word to act, especially as these sites are consulted by people with suicidal ideation. In the most recent study by Sakarya, Güneş and Sakarya (2013), a corpus of 100 webpages, built by entering five keywords into Google, is analyzed by three psychiatrists; the percentage of websites classified as "pro-suicide" is higher (40 per cent), and the authors insist that numerous sites have ambivalent content.

These different studies do not specifically address online discussion, but two of them (Cheng et al., 2011 and Biddle et al., 2008) emphasize that "pro-suicide" spaces are most often personal blogs and forums that are well-ranked. This is also the case for Wikipedia, the collaborative platform, which offers a very detailed page on ways to commit suicide, and which is often consulted for information on suicides (Biddle et al., 2008).

The content that Internet users are exposed to varies substantially, depending on which keywords are entered into search engines. Wong et al. (2013) also conducted a study intended to identify which pages are actually consulted by individuals making queries including the word "suicide". They identified 1,314 webpages, and then they examined the keywords used by people who visited these sites. The study shows that webpages accessed by individuals who enter queries including the word "suicide" are rarely websites that promote suicide (2 out of 1,314 webpages), with forums making up 2.3 per cent of these pages. Wong also stresses that the queries entered by Internet users to access suicide glorification websites do not necessarily include the word "suicide," but often refer to methods for suicide and their effects.

Several studies have examined the type of content featured on "pro-suicide" sites, including forums, highlighting that suicide is presented as an acceptable solution to problems in life, and is above all a personal choice, related to personal freedom (Durkee et al., 2011). Many of these sites call into question psychiatric approaches (Becker & Schmidt, 2005), and some stem from a counterculture that glorifies those "heroes" who affirm their choice by putting it into practice (Westerlund, 2011). "Pro-suicide" websites also offer a wide range of practical information on methods for "committing suicide well" or pain-free suicides, propose appropriate or original locations for the deed, and provide a considerable amount of information, often very scientific, on the effects of each method, whether they involve weapons or substances, with rather morbid, sometimes humorous descriptions. Pictures are occasionally included (Durkee et al., 2011; Westerlund, 2011; Alao et al., 2006). These websites also include advice for writing suicide notes, and sometimes even feature photos of suicide notes or death certificates proving that an individual has taken action, in addition to stories about celebrity suicides (Biddle et al., 2008). Some of these platforms seem to be used to create suicide plans (Becker & Schmidt, 2005) and are frequented by individuals looking for partners to make the deed easier, so that they don't "die alone" (Ozawa-de Silva, 2008). These suicide pacts have been primarily documented in Japan (Ozawa-de Silva, 2008; Lee, Chan & Yip, 2005; Rajagopal, 2004).

The content of sites that focus on prevention are less documented, except those that focus on actively preventing suicide. Many of these were created by institutions, community organizations and other individuals or groups of individuals affected by this problem. These pages generally give participants a chance to express their pain, to put it into words, often in the form of poems or literary texts, and to interact with peers who have lived through or are currently experiencing similar problems (Ozawa-de Silva, 2008). In some cases, they provide information on professional resources, allowing users to evaluate their risk of suicide through short questionnaires; some intervention sites give users the chance to talk online with a volunteer or professional responder (Barak, 2007), while other organizations have a presence on social networking sites like Facebook (Boyce, 2010).

An examination of the research analyzing the content available online and in discussion forums shows the great variety of content that can be found, but does not provide a very clear picture of the information that Internet users encounter, partially because content seems to vary for the different geographical zones studied, the keywords used in queries (and probably the Internet user's search history, which is used by search engines) and the time period studied, as the types of resources available online change quickly. Moreover, categorizing online content that appears in search engine results is not always easy, as some resources may be ambivalent, and it is impossible to predict their effects on the Internet users consulting them.

Effects of participation in online discussions about suicide on suicidal ideation

Qualifying and quantifying the impact that forums and chat rooms about suicide have on people in existential distress is quite difficult. It is important to first define "participation," as the effects are undoubtedly different if the Internet user contributes to the discussions or simply reads them. The literature on forums and chat rooms, excluding social networking sites like Facebook, emphasizes that the vast majority of users do not actively contribute, no matter what topics are discussed (Thoër, 2012). It is likely that this low participation rate also occurs in suicide discussion forums and chat rooms, though this remains unproven.

Furthermore, the effect of participating in online discussions remains poorly understood, especially since few epidemiological studies have been conducted. Most authors conclude that the Internet's effect is paradoxical: on one hand, participating in online discussion forums and chat rooms increases suicidal ideation and acting upon suicidal thoughts, but on the other, it allows individuals in distress to find resources and develop coping mechanisms, reducing the risk of suicide (Durkee et al., 2011).

Those who emphasize the negative effects of the Internet insist that using online discussion forums and chat rooms allows individuals to access information on how to commit suicide, helping to make their plans a reality by removing barriers to action (Harris, McLean & Sheffield, 2009). For example, Becker et al. (2004) analyzed a suicide attempt by a seventeen-year-old girl, revealing that she had visited online forums, chosen a method that was being discussed at that time, and obtained the substance used in her attempt from an anonymous poster whom she had contacted. Peer pressure could also encourage users to act. If they have announced their suicide plans online, these posters would feel pressured to act on their plans in order to avoid losing face, as discussions on these platforms can sometimes be very aggressive (Westerlund, 2011). This contagion effect is also highlighted in studies on suicide pacts (Takahashi et al., 1998; Lee et al., 2005). Finally, it is possible that people participating in online discussion are at greater risk (already have suicidal ideation or have made previous attempts). Dunlop, More and Romer (2011) show that increased suicidal ideation can be traced to exposure to suicide stories in forums, emphasizing that the most vulnerable youth in their study often participated in online discussions and blogs. It seems clear that participation does not have the same effect on everybody. McCarthy (2010) took the number of queries entered into Google for the terms "suicide" and "teen suicide" and linked them to the number of suicides reported by the U.S. Center for Disease Control. For all ages, he noticed an inverse correlation between the volume of searches conducted and the number of suicides reported, which could be explained by the fact that most people use the Internet to look for help, even if their initial participation isn't identified as such. The author observed, however, that in youth aged 15 to 25, the correlation was positive, with the number of searches for these key words increasing in parallel with the number of suicides reported, which seems to suggest that younger people are more at risk.

Sueki and Eichenberg (2012) also focus on the variable effects that participating in forums about suicide can have, based on participants' profiles and motivations. These authors have identified three participant profiles: those who register looking to help and to be helped, participants who are more ambivalent and are looking for all kinds of information on suicide (perhaps as preparation), and finally, those who have no clear motivation. If participating in these forums does not seem to aggravate suicidal ideation, regardless of the person's profile, the beneficial impacts would be more substantial for individuals looking for support than for those who are more ambivalent.

The beneficial effects of participating in online discussion for people experiencing existential distress would depend on the community aspect of these spaces and the possibility for participants to find help there. Participants in the 2008 study by Baker and Fortune, ages 18 to 30, were recruited from forums and chat rooms about suicide and self-harm; they said these spaces offered them a chance to interact with people who had similar experiences, were understanding, and didn't judge them. The anonymous nature of these sites also facilitated confessions about their troubles, which weren't always possible with loved ones and health professionals (Baker & Fortune, 2008; Winkel et al., 2005). Participation in online discussion about suicide, therefore, helped young people access credible information about similar experiences, practical advice that could easily be applied to their lives, and models (experience) for getting through these crises.

Participation in these communities also helped to reduce feelings of isolation and solitude, giving young adults a sense of belonging to a community, and in some cases, helping them build friendships (Baker & Fortune, 2008). Emotional support from these sites also seems to be linked to the fact that they validate the suicidal person's identity as such, which acts as a form of recognition and seems beneficial, though the strong sense of belonging to an online suicide community can also push participants to isolate themselves from the rest of society (Horne & Wiggins, 2009).

Studying interactions in online discussions about suicide

Many authors have examined the interactions that take place in online health discussion forums. These studies are conducted from a conversational and interactional perspective, intended to identify contribution methods (is it a testimonial, for example, or a cry for help, advice or information sharing?), norms for interacting and introducing oneself, the way that individuals use technology to communicate or introduce themselves, the way dialogue is structured and the roles participants play, and finally the information shared that the types of knowledge put to use (Thoër, 2012; Marcoccia, 2012). Our study on forums where young adults discussed using medication for other reasons than its intended purpose, in order to experience new sensations, illustrates the roles played by some contributors who express themselves more than others and act as experts within these sites (Thoër & Millerand, 2012). These users are characterized by specific types of contributions: they answer questions, supporting their contributions with personal experiences and scientific knowledge that they largely tend to have a monopoly on. They sometimes contribute to the forum's activity, acting as a type of memory bank, not hesitating to return to older messages and discussion threads. Finally, they offer support and encouragement to their peers and are more comfortable expressing their disagreement when actions discussed seem excessive, thereby contributing beyond their advice and comments to regulating practices.

There are quite few studies focused on the interactions that take place in forums about suicide. Horne and Wiggins (2009) analyzed two forums, selected for their high volume of traffic and the fact that accessing discussions did not require registration, and discovered several patterns in the forms of contributions and narratives presented. One of the patterns unfolds as follows: in a first message, the users establish their suicidal intentions and then explain that suicide is a logical solution to an unsolvable problem. This establishes the participant's suicidal identity. The authors also note that the authenticity of this status is primarily based on experience and the narration of this experience, not by a confirmed clinical diagnosis. Users therefore seem to favour an alternative approach, distancing themselves from biomedical discourse, as forums validate a different definition of existential distress.

The authors identified another pattern that would be categorized as seeking help. In this type of post, the users announce their intentions to commit suicide immediately and provide more or less specific reasons for ending their life. This type of post generally receives empathetic responses from others, who, for example, suggest that the person threatening suicide continue writing whatever they are thinking.

The authors saw that experience (having been there) is what gives posters some credibility, helping them give advice to others. One might wonder if this would also apply to forums focused on methods for committing suicide, in which some participants seem to distinguish themselves by showing their extensive technical, quasi-scientific knowledge of methods for killing oneself.

We do not know of any other studies that have analyzed interactions on suicide discussion forums, but the rich results presented by Horne and Wiggins (2009) illustrate the potential that these approaches have for better understanding the ways that these spaces are utilized and the influence that participants can have on one another.

Avenues for future research and intervention

Online discussion about suicide, and forums in particular, seem to act as spaces for expressing existential distress and providing aid and support, as well as offering information on methods for committing suicide and organizing suicide pacts. The effect that participating in these sites has on suicidal ideation and acting on suicidal thoughts is still poorly understood, due to a lack of epidemiological studies; however, these sites seem generally more preventative in nature, though variations seem to exist depending on the motivations and psychological states of participants. This is also apparent in research conducted on websites dealing with other at-risk behaviours, such as self-harm (Rodham et al., 2007; Murray & Fox, 2006), eating disorders (Borzekowski et al., 2010; Brotsky & Giles, 2007; Fox et al., 2005), or using drugs and medication in search of new sensations (Thoër & Millerand, 2012; Thoër & Aumond, 2011; Tackett-Gibson, 2007, 2008). These studies emphasize that these spaces contribute to the spread, normalization and acceptance of these practices as commonplace, in some cases encouraging continued commitment to these practices. These spaces also offer resources for managing risk. For example, a site will insist on the importance of taking low doses of medication in recreational settings in order to ensure comfort and enjoyment. These studies also show that these spaces allow participants to form bonds, receive emotional support and access resources that might not necessarily be easily available to them offline.

In terms of studies focused on online discussion about suicide, there are several limits, acknowledged by the authors. These include selection biases for the sites analyzed (choice of keywords entered into search engines, selecting forums that don't require the researcher to be a registered member) and, of course, users who agree to participate in surveys and qualitative studies, who are probably less at risk. Furthermore, evaluating the effects that participating in forums has on suicidal ideation is done retrospectively, after the user has already joined the forum. The results obtained about the nature of content available online, their use and their effects on suicidal ideation are therefore difficult to interpret, and it is especially difficult to generalize since the context of the forum depends on the content being shared. In order to describe the panorama of online discussion about suicide, it is important to conduct new studies that will analyze and compare content, identify the actors behind each of these sites and identify the specific content produced for the different types of social platforms used, as well as the links between these different spaces. Westerlund (2011) examined a pro-suicide forum, showing that it was linked to other spaces offering the same type of dialogue. We know that individuals rarely limit their search for information to a single site. Understanding how individuals and content circulate between these connected spaces will provide a clearer image of the social media space dedicated to suicide. Networking studies (Mercanti-Guerin, 2010) and virtual ethnography (Hine, 2000) offer new possibilities for dissecting the connected nature of online resources. In addition, while most of these studies focus on online communities for suicide, a large amount of information about health, and probably suicide, is also circulating on social networking sites like Facebook, where young people are quite active (Thoër, 2012). These sites would merit further attention.

Analyzing the online content relating to suicide that is available does not help us learn how individuals use it. It is therefore necessary to continue conducting qualitative and quantitative studies of active and passive users in these communities in order to better classify profiles of participants, their uses of the sites, and what participating in these sites means to them, as well as the effects this participation has on their suicidal ideation and suicidal behaviours. To this effect, longitudinal studies would be undoubtedly useful and easier to implement using online research methods.

It is especially important to better determine what is being said and what occurs in online discussions about suicide because social media grants users access to people's words and concerns as they are expressed, in a natural setting (Akrich & Méadel, 2002). This is especially important in instances of existential distress, as users who express themselves in social media tend to be younger and at greater risk, and do not seem to ask for help from traditional services (Horne & Wiggins, 2009; Barak & Miron, 2005). Analyzing these spaces also provides access to people expressing their suicidal ideation in a prospective manner, rather than a retrospective one (Horne & Wiggins, 2009), which offers an interesting opportunity for epidemiological surveillance and intervention (Page et al., 2011).

Finally, these spaces could become a source of inspiration for developing new forms of intervention (Barak & Miron, 2005). As Baker and Fortune (2008) have suggested, it may be that some of the people presenting suicidal ideation do not benefit as much from conventional interventions. Understanding what happens online and defining the role played by users who are identified as leaders or experts could be advantageous for developing new strategies for mutual assistance.

Conclusion

This chapter reviews the scientific literature in order to provide an analysis of the information about suicide that is circulating on social media, especially forums, as well as the effects that using these platforms has on suicidal ideation. These online dialogues about suicide seem to act as spaces for expressing existential distress and providing aid and support, as well as for offering information on methods for committing suicide and even organizing suicide pacts. The effect that participating in these sites has on suicidal ideation and acting on suicidal thoughts is still poorly understood. More research is clearly needed, including epidemiological studies. However, these sites seem largely more preventative in nature, though variations seem to exist depending on the motivations and psychological states of participants. This phenomenon is similar to what has been found by studies on spaces dedicated to other problems, such as self-harm, anorexia and use of medication in recreational settings. The methods chosen to interact about suicide with other users on social media platforms are not well documented. Analysis in other fields, however, suggests the potential that research on interactions could have, including developing a better understanding of the influence process and identifying leaders. Further study is therefore required to better understand the wide range of online content relating to suicide and the manner in which individuals use and appropriate this information.

References

Akrich, M., & Méadel, C. (2002). Prendre ses médicaments/prendre la parole : les usages des médicaments par les patients dans les listes de discussion. *Sciences Sociales et Santé*, *20*(1), 89–114.

—— (2009). Les échanges entre patients sur l'Internet. *La Presse Médicale, 38,* 1484–1490.

Alao, A. O., Soderberg, M., Pohl, E. L., & Alao, A. L. (2006). Cybersuicide: Review of the role of the Internet on suicide. *CyberPsychology & Behavior, 9*(4), 489–493.

Aubé, S., & Thoër, C. (2010). Construction des savoirs relatifs aux médicaments sur Internet : étude exploratoire d'un forum sur les produits amaigrissants utilisés sans supervision médicale, In L. Renaud, *Les médias et la santé: de l'émergence à l'appropriation des normes sociales,* Collection santé et société. Québec: PUQ, pp. 239–266.

Auxéméry, Y., & Fidelle, G. (2010). Impact d'Internet sur la suicidalité. À propos d'une "googling study" sur la rétro-information médiatique d'un pacte suicidaire échafaudé sur le Web. *Annales Médico-psychologiques, Revue Psychiatrique, 168*(7), 502–507.

Baker, D., & Fortune, S. (2008). Understanding self-harm and suicide websites. *Crisis: The Journal of Crisis Intervention and Suicide Prevention, 29*(3), 118–122.

Bandura, A. (1977). *Social learning theory.* Englewood Cliffs, NJ: Prentice- Hall.

Barak, A. (2007). Emotional support and suicide prevention through the Internet: A field project report. *Computers in Human Behavior, 23*(2), 971–984.

Barak, A., & Miron, O. (2005). Writing characteristics of suicidal people on the Internet: A psychological investigation of emerging social environments. *Suicide and Life-Threatening Behavior, 35*(5), 507–524.

Becker, K., Mayer, M., Nagenborg, M., El-Faddagh, M., & Schmidt, M. H. (2004). Parasuicide online: Can suicide websites trigger suicidal behaviour in predisposed adolescents? *Nordic Journal of Psychiatry, 58*(2), 111–114.

Becker, K, & Schmidt, M. (2005). When kids seek help on-line: Internet chat rooms and suicide. *Reclaiming Children & Youth, 13*(4), 229–230.

Biddle, L., Donovan, J., Hawton, K., Kapur, N., & Gunnell, D. (2008). Suicide and the Internet. *BMJ, 336*(7648), 800–802.

Borzekowski, D. L. G., Schenk, S., Wilson, J. L., & Peebles, R. (2010). e-Ana and e-Mia: A content analysis of pro-eating disorder web sites. *American Journal of Public Health, 100*(8), 1526–1534.

Boyce, N. (2010). Pilots of the future: Suicide prevention and the Internet. *The Lancet, 376*(9756), 1889–1890.

Brotsky, S., & Giles, D. (2007). Inside the "pro-ana" community: A covert online participant observation, *Eating Disorders, 15*(2), 93–109.

Buhi, E. R., Daley, E. M., Fuhrmann, H. J., & Smith, S. A. (2009). An observational study of how young people search for online sexual health information. *Journal of American College Health, 58*(2), 101–111.

Cheng, Q., Fu, K.-W., & Yip, P. S. F. (2011). A comparative study of online suicide-related information in Chinese and English. *The Journal of Clinical Psychiatry, 72*(3), 313–319.

Chou, W.-Y. S., Hunt Y. M., Burke Beckjord, E., Moser, R. P., & Hesse, B. W. (2009). Social media use in the United States: Implication for health communication. *Journal of Medical Internet Research, 11*(4), e48.

Dunlop, S. M., More, E., & Romer, D. (2011). Where do youth learn about suicides on the Internet, and what influence does this have on suicidal ideation? *Journal of Child Psychology and Psychiatry, 52*(10), 1073–1080.

Durkee, T., Hadlaczky, G., Westerlund, M., & Carli, V. (2011). Internet pathways in suicidality: A review of the evidence. *International Journal of Environmental Research and Public Health, 8*(10), 3938–3952.

Eysenbach, G., (2008). Medicine 2.0: Social networking, collaboration, participation, apomediation, and openness », *Journal of Medical Internet Research, 10*(3), Retrieved on 10 October 2009 from www.jmir.org/2008/3/e22/.

Fox, S., & Duggan, M. (2013). Health online 2013. Pew Internet and American Life Project, Washington, D.C. Pew Research Center. Retrieved 15 December 2012 from http://pewinternet.org/Reports/2013/Health-online.aspx

Fox, S., & Jones, S. (2009). *The social life of health information. Pew Internet & American Life Project* (p. 72).Washington, D.C.: Pew Research Center.

Fox, N., Ward, K., & O'Rourke, A. (2005). Pro-anorexia, weight-loss drugs and the Internet: An "anti-recovery" explanatory model of anorexia. *Sociology of Health and Illness, 27*(7), 944–971.

Gray, N. J., & Klein, J. D. (2006). Adolescents and the Internet: Health and sexuality information. *Current Opinion in Obstetrics and Gynecology, 18*(5), 519–524.

Gray, N. J, Klein, J. D., Noyce, P. R., Sesselberg T. S., & Cantrill. J. A. (2005). Health information-seeking behaviour in adolescence: The place of Internet. *Social Science and Medicine, 60*(7), 1467–1478.

Harris, K. M., McLean, J. P., & Sheffield, J. (2009). Examining suicide-risk individuals who go online for suicide-related purposes. *Archives of Suicide Research: Official Journal of the International Academy for Suicide Research, 13*(3), 264–276.

Harvey, K. J., Brown, B., Crawford, P., Macfarlane, A., & McPherson, A. (2007). "Am I normal?" Teenagers, sexual health and the Internet. *Social Science and Medicine, 65*(4),771–781.

Health Research Institute (2012). Social media "likes" healthcare: From marketing to social business, PricewaterhouseCoopers. Retrieved 15 December 2012 from http://www.pwc.com/us/en/health-industries/publications/health-care-social-media.jhtml

Herbert, C. F., Rioux, C., & Brunet, A. (2012). Les usages d'Internet par les personnes souffrant de troubles de santé mentale. In C. Thoër, & J. J. Levy (eds), *Internet et santé, usages, acteurs et appropriation* (pp. 177–204). Collection santé et société. Québec: PUQ.

Hine, C. (2000). *Virtual ethnography.* London: SAGE.

Horne, J., & Wiggins, S. (2009). Doing being 'on the edge': managing the dilemma of being authentically suicidal in an online forum. *Sociology of Health & Illness, 31*(2), 170–184.

Lee, D. T. S., Chan, K. P. M., & Yip, P. S. F. (2005). Charcoal burning is also popular for suicide pacts made on the Internet. *BMJ: British Medical Journal, 330*(7491), 602.

Marcoccia, M. (2012). L'analyse des interactions dans les espaces de discussion en ligne sur la santé. In C. Thoër, & J. J. Levy (eds), *Internet et santé, usages, acteurs et appropriations* (pp. 333–354). Collection santé et société. Québec: PUQ.

McCarthy, M. J. (2010). Internet monitoring of suicide risk in the population. *Journal of Affective Disorders, 122*(3), 277–279. doi:10.1016/j.jad.2009.08.015

McDaid, D., & Park, A.-L. (2010). Online health: Untangling the Web, BUPA Health Pulse 2010, Retrieved 20 February 2011 from <http://www.bupa.com/healthpulse>..

Mercanti-Guerin, M. (2010). Facebook, un nouvel outil de campagne : Analyse des réseaux sociaux et marketing politique. *La Revue des Sciences de Gestion, 242*(2), 17–28.

Morey, Y., Eagle, L., Verne, J., & Cook, H. (2011). Deliberate self-harm in the South West: Setting a research agenda. Discussion Paper. South West Public Health Observatory, Bristol. Retrieved 2 March 2013 from http://www.swpho. nhs.uk/default.aspx

Murray, C., & Fox, J. (2006). Do internet self-harm discussion groups alleviate or exacerbate self-harming behaviour? *Advances in Mental Health, 5*(3), 225–33.

Niezen, R. (2013). Internet suicide: Communities of affirmation and the lethality of communication. *Transcultural Psychiatry, 50*(2), 302–322

Ozawa-de Silva, C. (2008). Too lonely to die alone: Internet suicide pacts and existential suffering in Japan. *Culture, Medicine, and Psychiatry, 32*(4), 516–551.

Page, A., Chang, S.-S., & Gunnell, D. (2011). Surveillance of Australian suicidal behaviour using the Internet? *Australian and New Zealand Journal of Psychiatry, 45*(12), 1020–1022.

Rajagopal, S. (2004). Suicide pacts and the internet. *BMJ British Medical Journal, 329*(7478), 1298–1299.

Recupero, P. R., Harms, S. E., & Noble, J. M. (2008). Googling suicide. *The Journal of Clinical Psychiatry, 69*(6), 878–888.

Renaud, L. (2012). Internet et la promotion de la santé. In C. Thoër, & J. J. Levy (eds), *Internet et santé, usages, acteurs et appropriations* (pp.133–150). Collection santé et société. Québec: PUQ.

Rodham, K., Gavin, J., & Miles, M. (2007). I hear, I listen and I care: A qualitative investigation into the function of a self-harm message board. *Suicide & Life-Threatening Behavior, 37*(4), 422–430.

Romeyer, H. (2008). TIC et santé : entre information médicale et information de santé, *Tic&Société*, 2(1), consulté sur Internet (http://revues.mshparisnord.org/ticsociete/index.php?id=365), le 10 octobre 2012.

Sakarya, D., Güneş, C., & Sakarya, A. (2013). [Googling suicide: Evaluation of websites according to the content associated with suicide]. *Türk Psikiyatri Dergisi = Turkish Journal of Psychiatry, 24*(1), 44–48.

Sueki, H., & Eichenberg, C. (2012). Suicide bulletin bard systems comparison between Japan and Germany. *Death Studies, 36*(6), 565–580.

Tackett-Gibson, M. (2007). Voluntary use, risk, and online drug-use discourse. In E. Murgiuia, M. Tackett-Gibson, & A. Lessem (eds), *Real drugs in a virtual world: Drugs discourse and community online* (pp. 67–82). Lanham: Lexington Books.

—— (2008). Constructions of risk and harm in online discussions of ketamine use. *Addiction Research & Theory, 16*(3), 245–257.

Takahashi, Y., Hirasawa, H., Koyama, K., Senzaki, A., & Senzaki, K. (1998). Suicide in Japan: Present state and future directions for prevention. *Transcultural Psychiatry, 35*(2), 271–289.

The Change Foundation (2011a). Using social media to improve health care quality. A guide to current practice and future promise. Part 1: Introduction and key issues in the current landscape, <http://www.changefoundation.ca/docs/socialmediatoolkit.pdf>, consulté le 25 février 2012.

—— (2011b). Using social media to improve health care quality. A guide to current practice and future promise. Part 2: Exploring two case examples and imagining

the future, <http://www.changefoundation.ca/docs/socialmediaguidepart2.
pdf>, consulté le 25 février 2012.

Thoër, C. (2012). Les espaces d'échange en ligne consacrés à la santé : de nouv-
elles médiations de l'information santé. *Internet et santé, usages, acteurs et appropriation* (pp.57–91). Collection santé et société. Québec: PUQ.

Thoër, C., & Millerand, F. (2012). Analyser un forum sur les médicaments utilisés
à des fins récréatives : enjeux éthiques et méthodologiques. *Revue Internationale
de Communication Sociale et Publique, 7*, 1–22. http://www.revuecsp.uqam.ca/
numero/RICSP_7_2012.php#num7_1

Thoër, C., & Aumond, S. (2011). Construction des savoirs et du risque relatifs aux
médicaments détournés dans les forums sur Internet. *Anthropologie et Sociétés*,
numéro spécial "Cyberespace et Anthropologie : transmission des savoirs et des
savoir-faire", *35*(1–2), 111–128.

Westerlund, M. (2011). The production of pro-suicide content on the Internet: A
counter-discourse activity. *New Media & Society, 14*(5), 764–780.

Whitlock, J. L., Powers, J. P., & Eckenrode, J. E. (2006). The virtual cutting edge:
Adolescentself-injury and the Internet. *Developmental Psychology* [Special issue],
42(3), 407–417.

Winkel, S., Groen, G., & Petermann, F. (2005). [Social support in suicide forums].
Praxis der Kinderpsychologie und Kinderpsychiatrie, 54(9), 714–727.

Wong, P. W.-C., Fu, K.-W., Yau, R. S.-P., Ma, H. H.-M., Law, Y.-W., Chang, S.-S.,
& Yip, P. S.-F. (2013). Accessing suicide-related information on the Internet: A
retrospective observational study of search behavior. *Journal of Medical Internet
Research, 15*(1), e3.

3
E-Therapies in Suicide Prevention: What Do They Look Like, Do They Work and What Is the Research Agenda?

Simon Hatcher

This chapter describes current e-therapies and their potential role in suicide prevention. It discusses the benefits and problems of e-therapies and uses the example of "The Journal" in New Zealand to show where e-therapies may fit into a national suicide prevention strategy. The chapter then looks at the evidence about the effectiveness of e-therapies and concludes by identifying a research agenda for using e-therapies in suicide prevention.

E-therapies definition

One of the problems in this area is defining e-therapies. E-therapies are considered to be a method of e-Health. One systematic review found 51 different definitions of e-Health, most of which incorporated the themes of technology and health (Oh et al., 2005). The World Health Organization defines e-Health as "the transfer of health resources and health care by electronic means. E-Health provides a new method for using health resources – such as information, money, and medicines – and in time should help to improve efficient use of these resources." Health Canada defines e-Health as "an overarching term used today to describe the application of information and communications technologies in the health sector. It encompasses a whole range of purposes from purely administrative through to health care delivery"; whilst Wikipedia says e-Health is "a relatively recent term for healthcare practice which is supported by electronic processes and communication".

For the purposes of this chapter e-therapies are defined as treatments delivered by computers in a health care setting, often on-line or by a mobile phone. Here "treatments" is used in a wide sense and can include prevention, assessment, screening and diagnosis, as well as treatments for specific conditions. Telemedicine, which extends the range of individual clinicians, and the use of email or text message, have been specifically excluded. However e-therapies may be used in addition to traditional face-to-face services. An alternative but pithy definition is the MeSH term used by Medline in indexing articles on this topic, "computer-assisted therapy" which is defined as "Computer systems utilized as adjuncts in the treatment of disease".

What do they look like?

One conception of e-therapies is that they serve to provide information which produces change. In terms of suicide prevention, this can be thought of as a form of community development to improve mental health literacy. There are many web-based examples of this. For example, the National Suicide Prevention Lifeline in the United States presents videos of survivor stories (http://www.suicidepreventionlifeline.org/GetInvolved/Gallery), and The Suicide Prevention Resource Center (https://www.facebook.com/SuicidePreventionResourceCenter) and the Native American Suicide Prevention Program provide information on Facebook (https://www.facebook.com/NASPORG). However, the main focus in this chapter is on computerized therapies explicitly designed to produce change.

There are several generations of e-therapies. The first were essentially books on-line which required the user to read a lot of text, but there was little integration with mobile computing, and interaction was restricted to entering the answers to questionnaires. An example of this is MoodGYM (https://moodgym.anu.edu.au), which is based on cognitive behavioural and interpersonal therapies and aims to help people manage depression and anxiety. MoodGYM was not designed explicitly for people with clinical levels of depression and anxiety. Users work their way through five interactive modules that teach cognitive behavioural principles. It has over 500,000 registered users worldwide and has recently been translated into Chinese.

The next generation of e-Therapies involved not just text but some video and more interaction with the computer than just answering questionnaires. Examples are Beating the Blues and SPARX. Beating the Blues (http://www.beatingtheblues.co.uk) consists of eight sessions and is based on cognitive behavioural therapy. Users complete some questionnaires, read some texts and watch videos of people who describe how they used some of the lessons from the course. SPARX (http://sparx.org.nz/) is a novel treatment for depression in adolescents and uses a game to teach young people the principles of cognitive behavioural therapy by asking them to complete a quest around a fantasy island where they have to overcome various challenges and fight off "nats" – negative automatic thoughts – along the way.

More recent e-therapies integrate with mobile phones and other smart devices. An example is the Sir John Kirwan Journal, which is part of the New Zealand government National Depression Initiative which came out of the Suicide Prevention Strategy. The project also uses social marketing ideas to make users aware of the site and to monitor usage. Adverts on TV by Sir John Kirwan encourage people to visit the website (www.depression.org.nz) where users complete the PHQ-9 (a self-rating scale for depressive symptoms). Users then progress through an on-line journal which consists of six lessons based on cognitive behavioural principles (mainly problem solving). Each lesson consists of a video from Sir John Kirwan discussing the lesson with an expert. Then there is a task in which users can link to text or email reminders where they also get a pre-recorded message from Sir John Kirwan. The Journal also links to a telephone help-line to supplement the on-line content.

To date most e-therapies attempt to use computers to replicate what is done face to face. However, recent work is beginning to focus on what computers can uniquely do. The next generation of e-therapies will feature virtual environments, monitored environments and "mobile therapists". Virtual environments are already being used to treat anxiety disorders, in part driven by the search for effective treatments of post-traumatic stress disorder in combat veterans. Other areas of focus include fear of flying, panic disorder, social phobia and arachnophobia. The disadvantage of virtual reality is that patients still have to travel to a facility where the technology is available to get treatment since the ability to create virtual reality environments at home is still in its infancy. This mitigates one of the advantages of e-therapies, which is their convenience for the user. An extension of virtual reality is the acting out of therapy in virtual space, such as Second Life. Another form of novel treatment is computerized home monitoring which is already available commercially (for example www.magen.ca). Here users set up home monitoring so that they can, for example, get feedback about what they eat, how much exercise they do and whether they take medication on time. This approach is part of the increasing trend in western healthcare to personalize medicine. One of the challenges with this approach is to determine what happens to the information and who has access to it. Similarly, personalized health monitoring is now available on mobile applications. This is an obvious source for novel therapies for depression where smart phones can assess sleep patterns, exercise and location and could integrate these measures into a novel personalized depression treatment package. Ultimately, the therapy could be modified for an individual based upon feedback from the user about what the person was doing or feeling with therapies optimized by a computer based on the computer learning what works for others with similar feedback – intelligent real-time therapy.

A key issue is how the various therapies fit into existing clinical pathways. Most of the studies to date have not addressed this question. For instance, e-therapies could be an answer to the problem of long waiting lists to see therapists – why wait to see a person when a self-help programme on a computer can do the same job? This generates novel thinking about new roles in the health system, such as creating e-case managers who coach people through self-help programmes. People who do not respond to computerized therapies could then see a professional. The use of computerized therapies also raises questions about how health professionals can use such treatments as part of face-to-face treatment and the likely need for specialized training in these areas.

What are the benefits of e-therapies?

The potential benefits of e-therapies are that they are convenient for users who can access the treatments from anywhere, at any time, without any waiting lists. The therapies can also easily be tailored for specific groups, and there is some evidence that minority populations prefer on-line treatments to seeing someone face to face. The other significant advantage of e-therapies is that they address workforce shortages and novel roles in the health system. What hasn't been demonstrated yet is the cost effectiveness of e-therapies.

What are the problems with e-therapies?

The first objection to e-therapies is that they reinforce inequalities because of access and language. Not everyone has access to computers or the Internet, and those who don't are those most likely to be in deprived areas at highest risk of mental disorders. For example, in Canada in 2009 one in five individuals did not have access to the Internet from any location, and 23 per cent of individuals did not have home Internet access (http://www.statcan.gc.ca/tables-tableaux/sum-som/l01/cst01/comm36a-eng.htm). A recent review of mental health trusts in the English NHS found that one in four did not have sufficient computers to provide a service for users and in about a quarter of trusts the bandwidth was not sufficient to allow access to computerized cognitive behavioural therapy sites (Andrewes et al., 2013). Also, only half the trusts allowed clinicians to directly support patients by email whilst they completed on-line courses. This argument is becoming less powerful as computer and mobile phone ownership becomes ubiquitous, but Internet connections in remote areas are often poor or expensive. There is also the issue of language: minority populations are underserved in e-therapies since, with a few notable exceptions, English is the dominant language. For e-therapies which do not rely on reading large amounts of text this may be less of an issue.

There are also issues around privacy and confidentiality of data that users put into e-therapies. Whilst the boundaries around confidentiality appear to be changing (for example what people will tolerate being accessed on their Facebook page) there is clearly a need to restrict access to personal health data that can be linked to a user.

A third difficulty is that e-therapies rapidly become outdated with evidence about their potential effectiveness lagging about five years behind their development. This means that by the time e-therapies are used, they look and feel old compared to other commercial applications. There is also the problem of knowing when to retire old e-therapies as the platforms for which they were developed become obsolete.

Lastly, e-therapies are seductive, especially for researchers and policy analysts who spend a lot of time sitting in front of computers. These groups are expert computer users and to a large extent interact with the world through computers. Delivering treatments through an attractively packaged computer programme can seem very compelling to them. It is easy to forget that most people do not necessarily have these skills or the same access.

Where could e-therapies be used in suicide prevention?

When thinking about suicide prevention, where should we target our efforts? Figure 3.1 is adapted from a systematic review of suicide prevention strategies (Mann et al., 2005) and provides a useful guide to potential areas for intervention. Areas where e-therapies could potentially be of use are in education programmes for the general public (A); improving

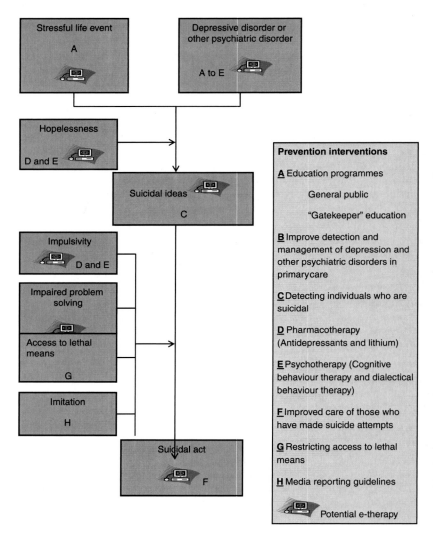

Figure 3.1 Targets of suicide prevention interventions and the place of e-therapies

the detection and management of depression and other psychiatric disorders in primary care (B); specifically targeting suicidal ideas (C); and delivering effective psychotherapies to those with psychiatric disorders or who have made a suicidal act (E and F).

An example from New Zealand is the National Depression Initiative which was linked to the National Suicide Prevention Strategy. Within the strategy, one of the areas identified where efforts should be made is in the better detection and management of depression in primary care. To break down the barriers to people getting help for mental disorders, a campaign, "Like Minds Like Mine," had already been in progress. This campaign used celebrities and consumers to talk about mental illness and to front an advertising campaign. Using this as a base, the National Depression Initiative developed a series of interventions to improve the recognition and treatment of depression. The initiative consisted of several components including a web site (www.thelowdown.co.nz) which specifically targeted youth with information about depression, the production of guidelines for General Practitioners about the treatment of depression in primary care and the creation of a self-help treatment programme for people with mild to moderate depression (www.depression.org.nz). This website was hosted by a celebrity, Sir John Kirwan, a rugby player who has spoken about his troubles with managing depression and anxiety especially when he was playing elite-level sport. Sir John Kirwan appeared in several TV adverts which referred people to the website where people could find more information about depression and could enrol in a self-help cognitive behavioural programme for depression, "The Journal". The Journal consisted of six lessons and used video to deliver information. The aim was to teach users problem-solving skills, which meant they had to create action plans which required a commitment to do things. Reminders to do the specific tasks that people had chosen to do were automatically emailed or texted to the user along with a pre-programmed message from Sir John Kirwan. The website also featured a phone help-line run by counsellors trained in problem solving that users could access if they wished. After the first year 700,000 people had accessed the web site, 20,000 people had registered with The Journal and there were 13,200 active users (Figure 3.2).

One of the noticeable features of tracking usage through The Journal is that whilst 13,020 people started, there is a large drop off in usage so that only 650 (5 per cent) completed all six lessons. This has been noted with other open-access web-based e-therapies. The responses to this are twofold: First, there is also a significant drop off with face-to-face therapies with most people not completing all planned sessions. The second response is that it may not matter as most of the improvement occurs in the first two or three sessions. For The Journal, the mean PHQ-9 score at start is 16, which decreased to 10 after two sessions and to 7 after six sessions among those who complete the programme.

Journal lesson activity

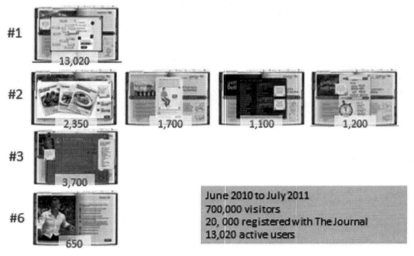

Figure 3.2   The Journal (www.depression.org.nz) usage activity

Of the people who completed the programme in the first year, 90 per cent showed some improvement, with 3 per cent not changing and 7 per cent indicating worse scores on the PHQ-9 than when they stared. Another noticeable feature is that about half the calls to the help-line were concerning technical issues of accessing or working through the computer programme. When users were surveyed about their reasons for not completing all six lessons, the most common reason given was "not had time" (45 per cent of responders), followed by "needed more support to keep going" (38 per cent) and "satisfied with what they had got" (32 per cent). This indicates that the website needs to be simple to use without time-consuming login procedures and that the provision of personalized support, perhaps by coaching with "e-case managers," may be a useful approach in the future. Although the website is marketed as a self-help programme for mild to moderate depression, primary care workers were encouraged by articles in the medical press to also refer people to the programme. When primary care workers were surveyed about the appeal of integrating The Journal into clinical practice, the mean score on a four point Likert scale, from 1 = does not appeal to 4 = appeals a lot, was 2.9 with non-physicians more enthusiastic about using it compared to family physicians.

An issue with using e-therapies in the field of suicide prevention is how to respond if people self-identify as suicidal or do not respond to the e-therapy. With The Journal, the programme will automatically send out prompts urging the user to seek professional help if they identify as suicidal or if their scores on the PHQ-9 do not improve. People do not need to enter personal details to use the web site, and users are anonymous. This could be seen as an advantage in suicide prevention: given that at least 60 per cent of people who commit suicide do not have contact with mental health services in the year before death, providing an intervention which is anonymous and avoids the stigma of mental disorders could be seen as way of reaching suicidal individuals who do not use traditional mental health services. Moreover, there is a negative relationship between suicidal thinking and help seeking (Deane, Wilson & Ciarrochi, 2001). Whilst tracing email and IP addresses is possible, this will usually involve law enforcement agencies and can be time consuming. There is a need to balance people's privacy and confidentiality against the need to preserve life in someone who may be mentally unwell. This of course is not a situation that is unique to computerized therapies.

As well as focusing on the treatment of depression, an alternative target is to specifically address suicidal thoughts (see, for example, van Spijker et al., 2012) An Australian version of this intervention "Living with deadly thoughts" is currently recruiting participants for clinical trials (http://www.blackdoginstitute.org.au/public/research/participatei-nourresearch/livingwithdeadlythoughts.cfm). One such study from Australia (Watts et al., 2012) found that after using a six-session Internet cognitive behavioural programme in a primary care sample of depressed patients the prevalence of suicidal thoughts reduced from 54 per cent to 30 per cent (although there was no control sample). Also of note is that in the two trials of Internet cognitive behavioural therapy by this group between 23 and 33 per cent were excluded due to suicidal ideation.

Do e-therapies work?

There is evidence from systematic reviews that e-therapies are as effective as face-to-face therapies. A review of ten systematic reviews (search date February 2011) on the effectiveness of computerized cognitive behaviour therapy in treating depression found limited evidence for the effectiveness of MoodGYM, Beating the Blues and Colour your Life (Foroushani, Schneider & Assareh, 2011). This review also concluded that there was evidence that computerized packages reduced therapists' time per patient, that they were no less effective than therapist-led cognitive behaviour therapy, and that they were equally or less effective than bibliotherapy. A particular issue with computerized therapies is calculating the cost effectiveness of the interventions, as the information needed is often "commercially sensitive" and unavailable. Also, computerized cognitive behaviour therapies have been recommended by the National Institute for Health and Clinical Excellence for the initial treatment of mild to moderate depression.(National Institute for Health and Clinical Excellence, 2009). However, many of the studies on e-therapies in depression have been on non-clinical populations recruited from the Internet, and few if any studies have shown any superiority to face-to-face therapy.

What is the research agenda?

The research agenda needs to focus on the different levels of suicide prevention: community development, primary care and secondary care. In the community there needs to be research which asks what is the best way to develop mental health literacy, reduce stigma and improve capacity to respond to suicidal people. This may include the simple provision of information or using tools from social marketing to support "gate keepers" in the community. Other interventions may address the causes of suicide, for example by providing indigenous communities on-line tools to strengthen their connections with the past and each other.

There has been little focus on primary care and how computerized therapies can be integrated with primary care, which is where most suicidal people present. Here there needs to be work on how computerized therapies fit into the workflow of primary care and the potential for new roles in primary care to manage patients using e-therapies. Sophisticated decision support that learns from the experience of similar patients in the same practice integrated with current guidelines is a potentially fruitful area.

In secondary care decision support, more intense personalized computerized care, perhaps combined with home monitoring, offers an advance on what we are doing at the moment. We need to conduct randomized controlled trials that include an intention to treat analysis, report adverse effects and include an economic analysis. A key question that is yet to be addressed is where e-therapies fit into existing pathways of care. For example, one obvious use for e-therapies is for people on waiting lists. Trials are needed to see if offering e-therapies here is useful. More work is also needed to tease out the effective components by comparisons with self-help, placebos and therapist-delivered therapy and head-to-head comparisons of different e-therapies.

As in psychotherapy research, there is a need to understand the processes that make e-therapies acceptable and feasible to people who are suicidal. We need to better understand what minority populations prefer and how computers interact with people to produce a change in behaviour. As has already been noted, one of the issues with unsupported on-line therapies is to better understand why people drop out of treatment and what can be done about it. Clinicians will need training in the use of computerized therapies with patients, and we need to determine the best ways to incorporate e-therapies into routine consultations. Related to this are the ethical and practical issues of using e-therapies. What is acceptable to users when it comes to privacy if they identify as suicidal and what are the legal implications of working with suicidal people outside the clinician's (or computer's) home province or country?

References

Andrewes, H., Kenicer, D., McClay, C. A., & Williams, C. (2013). A national survey of the infrastructure and IT policies required to deliver computerised cognitive behavioural therapy in the English NHS. *BMJ Open, 3*(2), e002277. doi: 10.1136/bmjopen-2012–002277.

Deane, F. P., Wilson, C. J., & Ciarrochi, J. (2001). Suicidal ideation and help-negation: Not just hopelessness or prior help. *Journal of Clinical Psychology, 57*(7), 901–914. doi: 10.1002/jclp.1058.

Foroushani, P. S., Schneider, P., & Assareh, N. (2011). Meta review of the effectiveness of computerised CBT in treating depression. *BMC Psychiatry, 11*(131). doi: 10.1186/1471–244X-11–131.

Mann J. J., Apter, A., Bertolote, J., et al. (2005). Suicide prevention strategies: A systematic review. *JAMA, 294*(16), 2064–2074. doi: 10.1001/jama.294.16.2064.

National Institute for Health and Clinical Excellence (2009). Depression: The treatment and management of depression in adults (Clinical guideline 90). http://guidance.nice.org.uk/CG90.

Oh, H., Rizo, C., Enkin, M., & Jadad, A. (2005). What is eHealth (3): A systematic review of published definitions. *Journal of Medical Internet Research, 7*(1). doi: 10.2196/jmir.7.1.e1

van Spijker, B. A., Majo, M. C., Smit, F., van Straten, A., & Kerkhof, A. J. (2012). Reducing suicidal ideation: Cost-effectiveness analysis of a randomized controlled trial of unguided web-based self-help. *Journal of Medical Internet Research, 14*(5), e141. doi: 10.2196/jmir.1966

Watts, S., Newby, J. M., Mewton, L., & Andrews, G. (2012). A clinical audit of changes in suicide ideas with internet treatment for depression. *BMJ Open, 2*, e001558. doi: 10.1136/bmjopen-2012–001558

4

Reducing the Burden of Suicidal Thoughts through Online Cognitive Behavioural Therapy Self Help

Ad J. F. M. Kerkhof, Bregje A. J. van Spijker and Jan. K. Mokkenstorm

Introduction

Many people who struggle with suicidal thoughts do not receive adequate help, either because they don't look for help, or they don't discuss their suicidal ideation with their general practitioner (GP) or health care provider. Shame, hopelessness, fear of rejection, fear of being admitted to a psychiatric institution, believing in spontaneous recovery of the problem, wanting to handle the problem alone, believing that treatment will not be effective, thinking the problem is not severe, and fear of stigma, all these factors may play a role (Bruffaerts et al., 2011). As a result, suicidal thinking may not be targeted in GP contacts or in mental health care. Suicidal persons do, however, look for anonymous and confidential support through crisis hotlines and organizations such as the Samaritans. Anonymity and confidentiality are key issues in providing support to those people with suicidal ideation who for whatever reason don't disclose their suicidal worries to others in face-to-face interaction. Telephone and Internet services may be important in interrupting their suicidal development. The magnitude of the problem is enormous: the year-prevalence of suicidal thoughts is around 3 per cent in The Netherlands, and the lifetime prevalence is estimated to be 11 per cent. The burden of disease of suicidal ideation is considerable expressed in Disability Adjusted Life Years: about 166,500 years in full health are lost due to suicidal thoughts (a provisional estimate based on Dutch year-prevalence rates) (van Spijker et al., 2011).

Cross-national data from 17 countries estimated the overall lifetime prevalence to be 9.2 per cent, with considerable variability in prevalence within countries (Nock et al., 2008).

The Internet

The Internet provides opportunities for suicide prevention: raising public awareness, educating about warning signs, identifying high risk groups and encouraging them to seek help, for instance through self-testing, peer-to-peer support forums and support or therapy via e-mail or chat services. A small number of online suicide prevention initiatives that provide an integrated and interactive combination of such services confirm the need for online help and support, as indicated by their services numbers (Barak, 2007; Mokkenstorm, Huisman, Kerkhof & Smit, see Chapter 10 in this volume).

Self-help through the Internet

Online self-help can be described as a standardized psychological treatment that can be worked through independently at home. Online self-help can be offered with or without therapist support. Many studies have demonstrated the effectiveness of web-based self- help for mental disorders such as depression, panic disorder, general anxiety disorder, social phobia, and problem drinking (Andersson & Cuijpers, 2009; Andrews et al., 2010; Riper et al., 2007). There are also indications that online self-help can be cost-effective (Gerhards et al., 2010; Warmerdam et al., 2010). Recently, a study into an Internet Cognitive Behavioural Therapy intervention for depression showed a decrease in suicidal ideation (Watts et al., 2012).

Self-help for suicidal thoughts via the Internet

We developed an online Cognitive Behavioural Therapy (CBT) self-help intervention aimed at reducing the frequency and intensity of suicidal thoughts, tested its clinical effectiveness, acceptability, and cost-effectiveness. In this chapter we describe the rationale for the self-help course, demonstrate some of the content, present a summary of the results, and describe its delivery in daily practice of the Internet site 113Online in The Netherlands.

Rationale: suicidal worrying and rumination

Suicidal individuals are often tormented by ruminative repetitive thoughts such as:

I want to stop my terrible thoughts
Nobody loves me
I am unlovable
I cannot live alone
I have no future
My life has no meaning
I am better off dead
My children will be better off when I am dead
I can't stand my depression
When will this stop?
When will my misery end?
I cannot stand my thoughts anymore

These thoughts can become tormenting when rehearsed many times a day for many hours. The wish to stop consciousness can, itself, also become a repetitive, compulsive thought that is rehearsed up to 24 hours a day: I have to stop thinking, I have to stop thinking, I have to stop thinking, etc. The wish to stop these repetitive thoughts may evolve into one of the driving forces behind the suicidal act. Worrying and rumination can be conceived as accelerators that speed up the wish to stop thinking altogether (Lester, 2012). Excessive worrying is one of the proximal risk factors for suicidal behaviour, as many survivors testify. In the end, the continuous repetition of these statements becomes a compulsion that cannot be controlled anymore (for an overview of worrying and rumination as risk factors for suicidal behaviour see Kerkhof & van Spijker, 2011). One of the most frequently reported motives reported by patients after their attempted suicide is: "My thoughts were so unbearable that I could not endure them any longer." These thoughts frequently centre on hopelessness, helplessness, and distress tolerance (Rudd et al., 2001). In times of crisis these thoughts become obsessive intrusions that can keep clients awake for several nights. Suicidal patients attribute their sleeplessness and vital exhaustion to the impossibility of stopping these thoughts.

Rationale: clinical implications

Awareness of worrying and ruminative self-talk in suicidal individuals may provide new ways of treatment of suicidal ideation. Cognitive behavioural treatment approaches, such as Wells' (2006) meta-cognitive therapy for worry, applied relaxation and cognitive therapy for pathological worry (Borkovec, 2006) and cognitive behavioural treatment for intolerance of uncertainty (Robichaud & Dugas, 2006), have led to good progress in the treatment of pathological worrying and rumination. These approaches can be usefully adapted for treatment of worrying in depressed and anxious suicidal patients. Exercises fostering worry postponement, positive worrying, and distraction can be helpful in the treatment of suicidal ideation.

The CBT self-help intervention

Living under control

The intervention consists of six modules, each of which can be completed in one week. Each module starts by providing information, followed by a weekly assignment and several core exercises, all of which are considered to be essential in order to benefit from the intervention and are therefore recommended to complete. In addition, each module lists a number of optional exercises to choose from. Each module is provided with a number of frequently asked questions (FAQs). Consumers can pose new questions, and these are answered in a general way. Ideally, consumers spend at least 15 minutes twice a day to perform the exercises. The aims of the six modules are:

1. To gain control over suicidal thoughts: The worrisome, repetitive aspects of suicidal thinking are outlined. The exercises are aimed at reducing suicidal worrying.
2. To recognize and prevent upcoming emotional crises: How to tolerate seemingly unbearable feelings and thoughts. Exercises are aimed at regulating intense emotions in a crisis situation.
3. To identify automatic suicidal thoughts: The ABC model of Activating events, Beliefs and Consequences is explained. Exercises are aimed at identifying and challenging automatic suicidal thoughts.
4. To address common distortions in thinking in general and in suicidal cognitions in particular: Exercises deal with recognizing and changing suicidal cognitions.
5. To challenge negative thoughts by evaluating evidence for and against their validity: Exercises focus on formulating alternative thoughts in a more detailed and neutral way.
6. To raise awareness to the possibility of relapse: Attention is given to future disappointments and setbacks and how to prepare for those.

Exercises focus on making a relapse plan and on formulating a realistic picture of the future.

Excerpts from the first module

Suicidal thoughts may feel like they are self-protective

Suicidal thoughts often arise because you are feeling down, discouraged and unable to find a solution to your difficulties. Your future seems dark and you may feel that there is no help and that all hope is lost. Problems seem to have piled up and you don't see a way out. Keeping on living then may seem to be a worse alternative to dying. Death seems like the only option left. The possibility of escaping if things get too bad can be a reassuring thought. Suicide then can seem to be the only way to protect yourself from further disaster.

Worrying about suicide

Thoughts about suicide can occur frequently, ranging from a few times a day to many times throughout the day. Common thoughts are:

"What is the meaning of this life?"
"I don't have a future anymore"
"I can't live all by myself"
"Everything has failed"
"People are better off without me"

When these sorts of thoughts are repeated many times a day, they become tormenting instead of self-protective. The thoughts that seemed to be helpful are now too frequent. They can intrude into your mind when you are not wanting to think about them and cause you to worry even more. Your thoughts can become so tormenting you desperately want to stop them. However, trying to control these thoughts is difficult. You may find that the more you try to stop your thoughts the more they occur. This is just how the brain works, and it happens not just for suicidal thoughts, but for other thoughts as well.

… Sometimes thoughts can become so tormenting, that people think of suicide as a way to stop their thoughts about suicide! ("My thoughts drive me crazy" or "I have to stop thinking.")

Week – assignment: tallying

How often do you think about suicide? And how much time do you spend on it? You can find out how much time you dwell on these thoughts by keeping a tally of your thoughts about suicide on a daily basis.

Table 4.1 Daily record of suicide-related thoughts

Day	How often?	How much time?
Monday		
Tuesday		
Wednesday		
Thursday		
Friday		
Saturday		
Sunday		

... This week we propose that you keep track of the number of times and amount of time you spend thinking about suicide. Use a note pad or a workbook to record (tally) every time you think about suicide, or have a suicide-related thought. If this is the same thought throughout the day, tally it every time you think of it. Also try to estimate the amount of time you think about these suicidal thoughts. At the end of the day, add your thoughts up and fill the number, as in Table 4.1 on the website.

Worry time

As you know, it is almost impossible to just stop your thoughts about suicide and things in your life that upset you. Consequently, it may be better to accept that these thoughts will be there, but to manage the times when you think about them. Therefore, you might like to consider, from now on, setting a time or two to worry. Set yourself a time twice a day in which you allow yourself to think about things that upset you or that you feel hopeless about. The rest of the day, try to postpone your thoughts about suicide and other upsetting things until the next worry time.

... Schedule your worry time for fixed periods during the day: one in the morning and one in the evening. Choose your times carefully so you can worry without being disturbed. Use an alarm clock, or the alarm on your mobile phone, or an egg timer to indicate when 15 minutes has passed. During worry time, consciously allow yourself to think about suicide and related subjects, such as your anxieties or fears. Once the worry time is up, get up and go and do something else. The rest of the day, try to postpone your thoughts until the next worry time.

Excerpts from the fifth module

Counter thoughts

Up until now, you've read that the way you think about events affects the way you feel. Now that you've got a good idea of your automatic thoughts and thinking habits, you can start to change them. To do this, we use counter thoughts, which are basically more neutral and detailed versions of your automatic thoughts. Changing your thoughts using counter thoughts can influence your feelings, by making them less negative. They will express similar feelings but be less intense. For example, the thought "My whole life has been ruined" can be countered by thinking "Important things in my life didn't go as I would've liked them to". The content of both statements is similar, but the second one is more detailed and more neutral or balanced than the first.

... What is the use of using counter thoughts? Imagine saying to yourself at least one hundred times "My whole life has been ruined". How would you feel afterwards? Now imagine saying "Important things in my life did not go as I would have liked them to" one hundred times. How would this make you feel? Is there a difference?

... You'll probably notice that repeating the first statement makes you feel more sad and hopeless than repeating the second one. By using counter thoughts, you can influence your mood in a positive way and gradually distance yourself from your more negative thoughts.

... Below, pairs of statements are presented. Each pair consists of one negative thought and one possible counter thought (i.e., a more detailed and neutral one). Indicate for each pair which statement you prefer and why.

- My life is meaningless.
- Counter: I find some parts of my life worthwhile, but others less meaningful.

I prefer this statement because ...

- Some thoughts are negative and difficult to stop.
- Counter: My thoughts are driving me crazy.

I prefer this statement because ...

- I'll always feel depressed.
- Counter: In the future, I'll probably feel depressed now and then, but not the whole time.

I prefer this statement because ...

- I'll experience several difficult moments today.
- Counter: How am I going to make it through the day?

I prefer this statement because ...

Next, try to think of counter thoughts for the statements below. You can compare your counter thoughts with the ones we came up with. Keep in mind though that there are many possibilities, so if your answers don't match ours, it doesn't mean they're wrong!

- I cannot handle this life.
- Counter: Several problems have been difficult for me to bear (and I am feeling discouraged).

- My feelings of guilt are unbearable.
- Counter: Several feelings of guilt are difficult to bear.

- Life has been unfair to me.
- Counter: There are several events that I've experienced as being unfair.

- I don't ever want to feel lonely again.
- Counter: I hope I'll experience less feelings of loneliness in the near future.

Effectiveness

In a randomized controlled trial the self-help intervention was compared with a six-week waiting list condition. In total 236 participants were allocated to the intervention group or to a control condition. Severely depressed or acutely suicidal participants were excluded because they needed more intensive care. Participants in the control condition had access to an information website containing risk factors and warning signs, and the nature and possible causes of suicidal feelings. In both conditions participants were allowed and even encouraged to seek regular help with a GP and mental health care services as well. During the experiment participants in both conditions were monitored bi-weekly as to their level of suicidality, and in case of increased suicide risk a safety protocol was followed, including telephone calls with the participants and their GPs. Because of the safety protocol, the participants had to disclose their identity. The primary outcome measure was the frequency and intensity of suicidal thoughts. Secondary outcome measures were levels of depression, hopelessness, anxiety, worrying, quality of life and costs related to health care utilization.

The results showed a significantly greater decrease in suicidal thoughts among the intervention group. Effects were more pronounced for participants who completed at least three modules. The effect size was small. The results are described in full detail in van Spijker et al. (submitted). The effects were maintained at a three-month follow-up. Economic evaluation revealed that there were considerable cost savings for society per clinically significant improved participant (van Spijker et al., 2012).

Acceptability

Participants in general were positive about the self-help course: The majority reported that their suicidal thoughts had decreased during the study, and their levels of satisfaction were acceptable. On average they spent 15 minutes a day following the course and practising exercises. Reasons for non-adherence or attrition were: a high level of hopelessness at the start of the course, self-reported lack of energy or discipline, lack of time, recovery from symptoms, admission to a psychiatric hospital, or commencement of psychological treatment elsewhere. Six participants reported aggravated symptoms or feeling more troubled by their thoughts. There were no suicides during the experiment. Eleven participants attempted suicide, of which seven participants were in the control group and four in the intervention group. Suggestions for improvement included: more provision of personal feedback or guidance and better tailoring the course to individual needs.

Discussion

As this is the first study of web-based self-help for suicidal thoughts, the results cannot be compared directly to previous studies. There is one recent Internet CBT intervention study targeting depression that found a decrease in suicidal ideation (Watts et al., 2012). The results of our study accord with what may be expected based on previous results for face-to-face cognitive therapy for suicidality and for unguided web-based treatment for related disorders. Although unguided programs generally demonstrate lower effect sizes than guided ones, the unguided nature of this intervention was integral to the study. The rationale for developing an unguided programme was based upon our desire to facilitate implementation and dissemination of the programme for crisis centres that are understaffed and mostly run by volunteers, and for both developed and developing countries wherever there may not be sufficient manpower to provide moderation or guidance. However, when means are available, guidance could potentially be provided.

The study incorporated a safety procedure in which participants at risk were contacted and GPs were involved as an ethical condition for this trial. The exclusion of severe suicidality and severe depression was part of the safety precautions. However, relatively few respondents were excluded because they were severely suicidal, indicating that the study sample represents a fair share of the suicidal population.

A limitation is that no formal psychiatric diagnoses were available, as no diagnostic instrument was administered. Rationale for this transdiagnostic approach lies in the fact that suicidality, the primary target of the intervention, can be present in many different psychiatric disorders. This approach is also in line with the implementation goal of the intervention, that it should become available to people with suicidal thoughts in general, irrespective of the presence of a diagnosed disorder.

The outcomes of this project demonstrate that online self-help is a valid and acceptable way of reaching people who might not otherwise seek help and that the intervention may work as an adjunct to regular care for those who are willing and able to seek this form of help.

The major implication is that suicidal thoughts can be reduced through online self-help. It is clinically relevant and meaningful to sufferers to reduce the psychological distress and burden associated with suicidal thinking. Particularly for those who are reluctant to access regular mental health services, it is, from our perspective, better to have some form of help or support than none.

Implementation

Because of the positive results, the intervention is now available with therapist e-mail support via www.113Online.nl, a Dutch suicide prevention platform that provides a range of services, such as a telephone helpline, an online crisis chat service, online psychotherapy, a moderated peer-to-peer forum, and self-tests (See Chapter 10 in this volume). Also, an English version is now being developed at the Black Dog Institute (Living with deadly thoughts). Finally, the text of the website has been published as a self-help book (*Worrying about Suicide*, in Dutch), lacking of course the interactive features of the website intervention (Kerkhof & van Spijker, 2012).

Since completion of the trial, the intervention has been implemented in 113Online. Via the 113Online homepage, visitors can apply for the self-help course by filling out an intake form, thus establishing an initial interactive contact with one of the 113Online professionals. Currently, one year after implementation, the number of participants per month fluctuates between 30 and 40. Participants are advised to use professional guidance and support, they are offered up to three e-mail exchanges to support them with the material and exercises of the course. One out of eight participants uses the guidance facility, most of them seeking guidance only once during the course. As expected, a minority of participants completed the entire course: 10 per cent completed five or more modules; 5 per cent completed the entire course.

Based upon the content of the guidance exchange messages 113Online professionals receive, the general impression is that many participants find the course to be helpful even after only three modules. They report suicidal rumination to have subsided to a significant degree, and thus feel more "air" and less entrapped by their thoughts. They manage to think about suicide in a more distant and objective manner. They feel more in control of their suicidal thoughts, and have learned to "park" these thoughts temporarily. Many participants report the first two modules to be quite confrontational, especially the exercises to register the intensity, duration and content of their suicidal worrying.

The participants' feedback gives some indication as to why the course is often not completed:

- The course may be just effective enough even when discontinued after the initial modules, in which participants basically learn that their ruminations are thoughts that can be modified and controlled, and they should not be overvalued as completely sound and objective reflections of their rational mind, and therefore they are not to be taken seriously at all times. Having learned this basic lesson may make completion of the entire course less necessary.
- Some participants find the course too difficult and not appealing enough.
- Some participants switch to other forms of treatment and help.

To summarize: it is feasible and effective to implement the self-help course in the practice of online suicide prevention work, and it could be performed by different organizations all over the world. Offering guidance requires little professional effort and seems to enhance usage to a modest degree.

Conclusions

Embedding the intervention in an integrated online suicide prevention platform such as 113Online has the advantage that people can be referred to a more intensive or immediate form of support when needed. Although implementation is subject to local conditions and a similar online platform may not always be available, the authors would recommend that some form of guidance is provided to users of the course if implementation were to occur in other locations. The amount of guidance can be varied in frequency and intensity according to individual needs or available resources. Providing guidance may also impact on adherence to the intervention. Ideally, this intervention would be implemented alongside existing telephone-based suicide and crisis support hotlines, which already have the expertise and infrastructure required.

Summary

Web-based help can reach people who do not seek or receive adequate care due to attitudinal barriers such as low perceived treatment efficacy or stigma, or due to geopolitical barriers when living in a region where (face-to-face) mental health care is less available or accessible. In addition, it can be used as an adjunct to face-to-face treatment. Although this study's effect size was small, the worldwide reach of the web and the low costs of guided and unguided web-based self-help could enable it to contribute appreciably to many suicidal individuals surfing the Internet looking for help.

References

Andersson, G., & Cuijpers, P. (2009). Internet-based and other computerized psychological treatments for adult depression: A meta-analysis. *Cognitive Behaviour Therapy*, *38*, 196–205.

Andrews, G., Cuijpers, P., Craske, M. G., McEnvoy, P., & Titov, N. (2010). Computer therapy for the anxiety and depression disorders is effective, acceptable and practical health care: A meta-analysis. *PLoS ONE*, *5*(10), e13196.

Barak, A. (2007). Emotional support and suicide prevention through the Internet: A field project report. *Computers in Human Behavior*, *23*(2), 971–984.

Borkovec, T. D. (2006). Applied relaxation and cognitive therapy for pathological worry and generalized anxiety disorder. In G. C. L. Davey & A. Wells (eds), *Worry and its psychological disorders: Theory, assessment and treatment* (pp. 273–288). Chichester: John Wiley & Sons, Ltd.

Bruffaerts, R., Demytenaere, K., Hwang, I., Chiu, W. T., Sampson, N., Kessler, R. C., et al. (2011). Treatment of suicidal people around the world. *British Journal of Psychiatry*, *199*, 64–70.

Gerhards, S. A. H., de Graaf, L. E., Jacobs, L. E., Severens, J. L., Huibers, M. J. H., Arntz, A., et al. (2010). Economic evaluation of online computerised cognitive-behavioural therapy without support for depression in primary care: randomised trial. *British Journal of Psychiatry*, *196*(4), 310–318.

Kerkhof, A. J. F. M., & van Spijker, B. A. J. (2011). Worrying and rumination as proximal risk factors for suicidal behaviour. In R. C. O'Connor, S. Platt & J. Gordon (eds), *International Handbook of Suicide Prevention: Research, Policy and Practice* (pp. 199–209). Chichester: Wiley – Blackwell

Kerkhof, A. J. F. M., & van Spijker, B. A. J. (2012). *Worrying about suicide* (in Dutch). Amsterdam: Boom.

Lester, D. (2012). The role of irrational thinking in suicidal behavior. *Comprehensive Psychology*, *1*(8), 1–9.

Nock, M. K., Borges, G., Bromet, E. J., Alonso, J., Angermeyer, M., Beautrais, A., et al. (2008). Cross-national prevalence and risk factors for suicidal ideation, plans and attempts. *British Journal of Psychiatry*, *192*, 98–105.

Riper, H., Kramer, J., Smit, F., Conijn, B., Schippers, G., & Cuijpers, P. (2007). Web-based self-help for problem drinkers: A pragmatic randomized trial. *Addiction*, *103*, 218–227.

Robichaud, M., & Dugas, M. J. (2006). A cognitive behavioral treatment targeting intolerance of uncertainty. In G. C. L. Davey, & A. Wells (eds), *Worry and its psychological disorders: Theory, assessment and treatment* (pp. 289–304). Chichester: John Wiley & Sons, Ltd.

Rudd, M. D., Joiner, T. E., & Rajab, M. R. (2001). *Treating suicidal behavior: An effective, time-limited approach.* New York: The Guilford Press.

van Spijker, B. A. J., Majo, C. M., Smit, F., van Straten, A., & Kerkhof, A. J. F. M. (2012). Reducing suicidal ideation: Cost-effectiveness analysis of a randomized controlled trial of unguided web-based self-help. *Journal of Medical Internet Research*, *14*(5), e141.

van Spijker, B. A. J., van Straten, A. Kerkhof, A. J. F. M. (submitted). Effectiveness of online self-help for suicidal thoughts: Results of a randomised controlled trial.

van Spijker, B. A. J., van Straten, A., Kerkhof, A. J. F. M., Hoeymans, N., & Smit, F. (2011). Disability weights for suicidal thoughts and non-fatal suicide attempts. *J Affect Disorders*, *134*, 341–347.

Warmerdam, L., Smit, F., van Straten, A., Riper, H., & Cuijpers, P. (2010). Cost-utility and cost-effectiveness of Internet-based treatment for adults with depressive symptoms: Randomized trial. *Journal of Medical Internet Research*, *12*(5), e53.

Watts, S., Newby, J. M., Mewton, L., & Andrews, G. (2012). A clinical audit of changes in suicide ideas with Internet treatment for depression. *BMJ Open*, *2*(5), e001558.

Wells, A. (2006). Metacognitive therapy for worry and generalised anxiety disorder. In G. C. L. Davey, & A. Wells (eds), *Worry and its psychological disorders: Theory, assessment and treatment* (pp. 259–272). Chichester: John Wiley & Sons, Ltd.

5

Challenges in the Control and Regulation of Suicide Promotion and Assistance over the Internet

Brian L. Mishara and David N. Weisstub

There has been growing concern about the numerous case-reports of suicides following contact with Web sites that incite people to suicide and provide detailed information on suicide methods (Alao, Yolles & Armenta, 1999; Australian IT, 2004; Baume, Cantor & Rolfe, 1997; Becker & Schmidt, 2004; Dobson, 1999; Luxton, June & Fairall, 2012; Mehlum, 2000; Niezen, 2013; Rajagopal, 2004; Reany, 2004; Richard, Werth & Rogers, 2000; Robertson et al., 2012; Thompson, 1999). This article presents and discusses ethical, legal and practical issues in the control and regulation of suicide promotion and assistance over the Internet.

There are numerous reports in the media and scientific journals of suicides purportedly related to contact with Internet sites. Typical examples include the suicide, which instigated the introduction of a bill in the Danish Parliament in February 2004 to ban websites that encourage and provide information about suicide. The son of a Danish journalist was apparently encouraged to end his life by a website that gave him information he used to kill himself. Becker and colleagues (Becker, El-Faddagh & Schmidt, 2004; Becker et al., 2004), who reported on a 17 year old female suicide attempter, concluded that Web sites may trigger suicidal behaviour in pre-disposed adolescents. Several newspaper articles tell of distraught parents who blamed their child's suicide on Internet sites (Shepherd, 2004).

The Internet may glorify suicides by ensuring the attention of multiple onlookers. For example, in 2008, the suicide of a young man was broadcast using a webcam over the Internet while 1,500 people apparently watched as the man lay dying (Polder-Verkiel, 2012). When someone finally called the police, it was too late.

Multiple suicides by people who meet on chat sites appear to be increasing. A much-publicized example concerned Louis Gillies from Glasgow who met Michael Gooden from East Sussex (England), in May 2002, on a suicide "newsgroup" (Innes, 2003). While on a cliff ready to jump, Mr. Gillies was talked out of killing himself by a friend on his cell phone, but Mr. Gooden refused to talk and jumped. Mr. Gillies was charged with aiding and abetting a suicide; he killed himself in April 2003, just before the trial was about to begin.

Meeting suicide companions online appears to be most prevalent in Japan (Japon, 2004) where, between February and early June 2003, at least twenty Japanese died in suicide pacts with companions they met on the Internet, many by strikingly similar carbon monoxide poisonings (Harding, 2004; "Seven die", 2004). It is believed that the first "wave" of Internet suicide pacts occurred in 2000 in South Korea when there were three cases. In March 2003, an Austrian teenager and a 40-year-old Italian who met on a suicide chat jointly committed suicide near Vienna ("Pair planned suicide", 2003). The man had also contacted two young Germans via online chat, but Police alerted their families before they could carry out their suicides.

Legal provisions and law reform projects

Many countries have laws prohibiting aiding and abetting suicide; however, we are not aware of any case where Internet activity has been pursued in a court of law for aiding or abetting suicide. However, on 13 February 2005, Gerald Krein was arrested in Oregon for solicitation to commit murder after it was alleged that he used his Internet chat room to entice up to 31 lonely single women to kill themselves on Valentine's Day. The arrest followed a report to police by a woman in the chat room who said another participant talked about killing her two children before taking her own life (Booth, 2005). We may wonder why current laws against aiding and abetting suicide have not been applied to Internet activities, given the compelling nature of specific case histories when people died by suicide in a manner communicated over the Internet and following a series of Internet contacts in which they were encouraged to kill themselves.

It may be helpful to examine legal jurisprudence regarding standards for determining causality in such matters. When individuals are deemed to be responsible for having caused harm to another person, their actions are usually in close temporal and physical proximity to the victim's death. For example, a person who strikes another person who subsequently dies from the blow may be deemed to be responsible because that action had an immediate physical consequence for the victim. As well, scientific and medical evidence must indicate according to reasonable probabilities that the action in question was causally related to the consequences (Bonger, 2002).

Scientific evidence

Scientific research on the influence of the media on suicides has concentrated on television and newspapers and their influence on population suicide rates. There are several excellent reviews of research in this area (e.g. Hawton & Williams, 2001; Pirkis & Warwick Blood, 2001; Stack, 2000; 2003; 2005). It is clear that news media depictions of deaths by suicide have a risk of increasing suicides among those who have contact with those media. Generally, the more the publicity, the higher the contagion effect. It has been reported that the suicide of Marilyn Monroe resulted in 197 additional suicides (Phillips, 1974). However, there are no empirical data on changes in the risk of suicide that may be related to contacts with Internet sites. Nevertheless, it appears from numerous cases reported in the media that contact with Internet sites and with chat rooms preceded deaths by suicide and the methods used were precisely those described in the Internet contact. In sum, these case reports do not meet the requirements for scientific proof that Internet sites cause suicide, but they suggest that a relationship may exist.

Despite the compelling case reports, it can be argued that had the victims not contacted a specific suicide site, they may have still killed themselves. The suicide risk of people who contact suicide sites may have pre-dated their contact. In addition, if a person had not used a method found on a site, other methods are easily available.

A recent study by Biddle and colleagues (Biddle et. al., 2012) reported the results of interviews with 22 suicide attempters in hospital asking where they obtained information about self-harm. Thirteen of the 22 respondents said that they sought information about suicide on the Internet before their attempt, and eight said that the Internet played a role in shaping their suicide plan, in several instances by providing concrete information on a suicide method.

A challenge in determining a causal relationship is the difficulty in generalizing from epidemiological population statistics to individual cases. According to population statistics, it has been demonstrated that media publicity on suicide results in a small but significant increase in the number of people who die by suicide following the media reports.

However, it is not possible to generalize from these population data to determine if any one specific individual's death was facilitated by his having read a newspaper article or having watched a specific television program about suicide. The nature of epidemiological research is such that, given the great number of people at risk of committing suicide and the very small number who actually die by suicide, it is impossible to determine that one specific individual is likely to have died as a result of media exposure and that the death could have been avoided by non-exposure. However, research may shed some light on the issue. An examination of the role of electronic communication, specifically online social networking and SMS text messaging, in an adolescent suicide cluster in New Zealand (Robertson et al., 2012) found that the cluster of suicides from students in different schools was associated with visits to social networking sites, including sites created in memory of suicide victims. The probability of observing the cluster of suicides so close in time and geographic location by chance alone was .009.

To date we have little epidemiological data on the relationship between contact with the Internet and suicides. All we have is a number of case histories in which there appears to be a link and some instances where suicide victims contacted websites before their attempts and used methods they found online. It is dubious that one could make a good scientific or legal case for the causal relationship between Internet activities and suicide without conducting further research.

Self-regulation

Even if one could prove that there is a risk associated with certain Internet sites, one must weigh the risk against possible dangers of compromising freedom of expression by attempting to control access to the site. In most countries, there is little or no control of Internet content because of constitutional guarantees of freedom of expression. The EU decision number 276–1999 "The European Union Safer Internet Plan" (European Union, 1999) essentially proposes that Internet organizations and Internet Service Providers (ISPs) act responsibly to control what is available and limit or deny access to sites that are illegal or dangerous. Many countries, including Great Britain, Canada, the United States and New Zealand, attempt to control Internet content by self-regulation since guarantees of freedom of speech apparently preclude censorship or government control of access to sites. The use of self-regulation has been criticized for being ineffective since those who produce the sites and distribute them are also being asked to censor them. It has also been criticized by persons who are concerned about the defence of freedom of expression. There is no verification of which sites are blocked or censored and no explicit guidelines about what should be banned.

Filtering techniques

An alternative to self-regulation is rating systems that use filtering techniques to block access to certain sites on personal computers. A primary issue is who actually rates the sites so that filter programs can identify sites to block. The World Wide Web Consortium (W3C) has developed the "PICS" standards in which creators of sites rate their own sites according to specific criteria. However, ratings of sites, even if accurate, are useless if they are disregarded. Software used to filter sites by blocking access is only effective if they are used and they block target sites and do not block other permissible sites. For this reason, filtering software is mostly used by parents who attempt to control access to sites by minors; for example, sites depicting child pornography, violence, and racial hatred. But filters have limited intelligence to discriminate between desirable and undesirable sites. If filters block access to certain words or terms, for example "suicide," or "suicide methods," they may also block sites that provide helpful information in suicide prevention, such as the site of Befrienders International, which offers help over the Internet to suicidal individuals (www.befrienders.org)

Blocking access to sites

A number of countries attempt to block access by all individuals to specific Internet content and sites, including Algeria, Bahrein, China, Germany, Iran, North Korea, Saudi Arabia, Singapore, South Korea, Sweden, United Arab Emirates, and Vietnam. For example, in Saudi Arabia all 30 of the ISPs go through a central node, and material and sites containing pornography, believed to cause religious offence and containing information on bomb making are blocked. Germany requests that ISPs block media that is morally harmful to youth including that which is "pornographic, depicts extreme violence, war mongering, racist, fascist or has anti-Semitic content". They have had success in blocking German sites with this material but have been less successful in blocking sites originating outside of Germany. Sweden has laws that require blocking of information instigating rebellion, racial agitation, child pornography, illegal description of violence, and material that infringes upon copyright laws.

In several countries, including the USA, England, and New Zealand, laws were passed to block other Internet content, but those laws were overturned by the courts because of constitutional guarantees of freedom of expression. Australia is the only country that currently has laws to specifically restrict sites that promote suicide or provide information on suicide methods.

Modifications to the Australian Criminal Code

Public concern about the vulnerability of Australian youth recently gave rise to the enactment of amendments to the Australian Criminal Code making Internet activity intentionally done, relating directly or indirectly to the incitement of suicide, as a distinct crime (Criminal Code Amendment (Suicide Related Material Offences) Act, 2005). The Australian legislation, which came into force in 2006, makes it a criminal offence to use a carriage service (Internet, telephone, television, etc.) to disseminate material intended to counsel or incite suicide. Also, providing instructions on how to commit suicide or promoting a specific method are illegal, as well as possession, production and the supply of such material.

The Parliamentary debate highlighted the vulnerability of young adults as a particular group based on both their level of Internet usage and their suicide rates (Commonwealth of Australia, 2004b; 2004c). It was argued that because of those factors there is a moral obligation on the part of society to provide protection. The legislators cited the failure of private ISPs to regulate themselves, thereby mandating government to do so. While acknowledging the division in public opinion, the Australian government argued that public protection trumped issues of liberty and freedom of expression.

Nevertheless, there was strong vocal opposition, including from the Green Party. The critiques said that the ambiguity of "intentionality" could give rise to unintended results and could render the law impossible to apply. The point was argued that given the volume of suicide items incorporated into daily activity on the Internet, it could be foreseen that ISPs could readily find themselves vulnerable to the legislation despite their efforts to control content if an aggressive pattern of catchments would take place. It was submitted that attacking the causes of suicide, rather than operating with a wide net of surveillance and intervention, would be more likely to succeed.

Other interventions addressed the foolhardiness of attempting to restrict information about matters such as suicide and voluntary euthanasia. The key issue, from the point of view of the opposition, was not the need to control Internet content, but rather, the extent to which the government is prepared to devote resources to suicide prevention activities.

Pirkis and colleagues (2009), in their assessment of the impact of the Australian legislation felt that although the law cannot effectively impact overseas web sites, the law has the potential to reduce access to domestic web sites and deliver substantial benefits in suicide prevention. Furthermore, they contend that regardless of the capacity of the law to limit access to pro-suicide sites, the legislation sends a clear message to people who would promote suicide: that this is not socially acceptable in Australia.

Ethical presuppositions

There are several ethical considerations concerning the control of Internet content in order to prevent suicide. First and foremost is the ethical premise that suicide should be prevented (Mishara & Weisstub, 2005). Those who adopt a libertarian perspective might contend that people have the right to choose to end their life by suicide. Also, since suicide is not illegal in most countries, it may appear that suicidal people should have access to material they desire. If one adopts this libertarian position, it is not possible to justify controlling access to information encouraging suicide or providing information or advice on how to exercise the right to end one's life by suicide.

If one adopts a moralist ethical position, then suicide must be prevented, and if controlling access to Internet sites can save lives, it must be instituted. If one holds a relativist position that some suicides are acceptable and others are not, one may morally justify some form of Internet control. However, control of access for only some people is practically impossible. For example, a relativist who believes that terminally ill people should be allowed or have access to means to end their lives but people in good health who suffer from treatable psychiatric problems should not, would have a difficult time controlling access for some people and not others.

The Internet versus other mass media

One of the questions concerning the ethics of controlling access to the Internet is the specificity of the Internet compared to other mass media. The Internet has been characterized as a "pull" technology, as opposed to the so-called "push" technologies including radio and television. Push technologies provide access to the media without the user engaging in any specific and explicit attempt to find a specific media content. Television content is available in every home, and because of its universal access, television has been regulated in most countries as to content. In contrast to the mass medias of television and radio, the Internet users must actively seek out specific content.

Also, anonymity of the provider can exist on the Internet, and there is no ability to verify the authenticity of the information one finds on a website. No government agencies are ensuring that web content is appropriate and accurate (unlike television and radio which are generally subject to government control). The Web can be extremely graphic in nature, and individuals who display their suicidal intentions and behaviours on the Internet can expect possible exposure to thousands throughout the world, providing glorification of their suicidal acts.

The differences between "push" and "pull" technologies may be used to defend the Internet against control by claiming that the Internet is a private matter which does not invade people's homes, but rather that specific content must be sought out by individuals actively searching through cyberspace. However, its nature also provides for a level of anonymity of both the person contacting the site and the person providing information on a site, which may lead to an "anything goes" environment where there are no controls whatsoever about the authenticity and credibility of information transmitted or provided.

Different Internet activities

Internet situations involving suicide vary. Some sites passively provide information that encourages suicide in texts that suggest it is a good idea to end one's life. Other sites provide information on suicide methods, many including specific details about what medications to mix, how to hang oneself, and the strengths and weaknesses of alternative methods with respect to side effects and risks of "failure". Other sites involve the exchange of messages from "suicide encouragers" who interact with suicidal people, trying to stimulate them to proceed with their suicidal plans in chat rooms or in e-mail correspondence. "Suicide predators" seek out people who post messages suggesting they may be feeling suicidal but who are not explicitly asking for information or encouragement. "Predators" offer unsolicited incitation to suicide and may provide information about how to commit suicide without being asked. If one is considering some form of control of Internet activity, it is important to decide which of the above activities one would like to limit.

Vulnerable populations

One of the major issues in control of the Internet in order to prevent suicides is the protection of minors and other vulnerable populations, such as persons with psychiatric disorders. The most successful attempts to control access over the Internet has involved child pornography sites and pornography aimed at minors, although these initiatives may be criticized for falling short of their goal of totally blocking access. However, very little has been done to protect minors from suicide promotion sites.

In the area of the exposure of minors to extreme violence, there are empirical data on possible negative effects, but little has been done to control access over the Internet. Research has shown beyond doubt that media exposure to violence is related to increased violent behaviour (Bushman & Anderson, 2001). However, there is little success in attempts to control violence on the Internet.

The jurisdictional factor

Even if one were able to resolve the legal and ethical issues, there are a number of practical considerations that make control of Internet suicide promotion activities extremely difficult (Geist, 2002; Smith, 2002). The first is the issue of cross-border jurisdiction. Although countries may be able to control activities of Internet sites that originate within their borders, international jurisprudence makes it difficult to obtain jurisdiction over Internet sites that originate outside the country. Jurisprudence generally distinguishes between passive Internet activity, such as simply operating a website which may be accessed from different countries, and active endeavours which involve sending information, interacting (for example, in a chat room) and doing business in a country. Furthermore, jurisprudence has favoured limiting claims of harm to actual impact rather than claims of potential damage.

Two important cases underline the difficulties in cross-border jurisdiction issues. The first case, in Canada, *Braintech Inc. v. Kostivk* (1999), involved a libel complaint concerning a site in Canada. In denying jurisdiction, the judge found that there is a "need for better proof the defendant entered Texas than the mere possibility that someone in Texas may have reached to cyberspace to bring defamation material to a screen in Texas." Just having material on a site outside a jurisdiction was shown to not be sufficient to allow for jurisdiction in another area (Geist, 2002).

The "Calder test," based on the U.S. case of *Calder v. Jones* (1984), is often used to determine jurisdiction in Internet cases. This test requires that: (1) the defendant's intentional tortuous actions are expressly aimed at the forum state and (2) causes harm to the plaintiff in the forum state, of which the defendant knows is likely to be suffered. This test provides protection for Internet sites and activities that do not explicitly attempt to have an effect outside of their own jurisdiction or intentionally cause harm to an individual in another jurisdiction. Obviously, there is virtue in protecting individuals from being liable in every country in the world for actions that may be perfectly legal in their own jurisdiction. Still, jurisdiction issues make attempts to control Internet activity extremely difficult.

Conclusion

There is a great need for scientifically valid data on the extent that Internet sites contribute to the risk of suicide. More specifically, we need to determine if Internet activities increase suicide risk and if so, which sub-populations are particularly vulnerable to being affected by the Internet. There are many spectacular media reports of suicides following Internet contact and case reports of individuals who died by suicide using methods they found on the Internet. There are increasing reports of pacts in which people met over the Internet and subsequently died by suicide. However, as impressive as these reports may seem, they do not constitute scientific proof that Internet activities provoke suicides. One could try to build a case for the relationship between Internet activities and suicide using psychological autopsy methods. Qualitative assessments of the content of Internet contacts where seemingly vulnerable individuals appeared to be forcefully encouraged to kill themselves have high face validity. However, we need to develop more creative methodologies, perhaps inspired by the studies of the relationship between suicide reporting in other media and suicide rates. One of the greatest challenges is to determine if individuals who kill themselves after Internet contacts would have died by suicide if they had not used the Internet.

It is also important to clarify the ethical basis upon which any form of suicide prevention activity is undertaken before applying one's beliefs to controlling Internet suicide promotion. Furthermore, any action to control Internet suicide promotion must consider the different forms of Internet activities, ranging from passive posting of information on a website to interacting in a chat room or seeking out vulnerable individuals as an Internet "predator".

Any attempt to control the Internet must be viewed in the perspective of the control and freedom of other media, unless special characteristics of the Internet are judged to lead to special laws or consideration. It can be argued that, unlike other media, the Internet lacks quality control and oversight, and this may justify legislative intervention. However, editors of newspapers, like webmasters, are free to publish what they please, even if it may incite suicides. If a journalist publishes a "dangerous" article, she may evoke the ire of readers and sales may decline (or increase due to the controversy). When a website or chat does something people do not like, users can simply not frequent that site. In this regard, it is interesting to compare the Internet to published works. If one were to publish the philosopher David Hume's writings recommending suicide on an Australian Internet site, could this be banned? If so, could it be considered as more dangerous than publishing his book and selling it in a bookstore? Internet sites provide information on means to kill oneself. However, if the same information is available in medical textbooks, what may justify controlling providing this information over the Internet while permitting the sale of medical textbooks and their availability in libraries?

The fact that the Internet allows for global access leads to complex jurisdiction issues and practical difficulties. Given the rapidly changing state of technologies, which lead to the continued development of new ways to circumvent control, it may not be practically possible to ban sites, censor material or limit access. Even if we had convincing data to document a high risk of suicide being related to specific Internet activities, and even if a country decides to prevent access to suicide sites, the only way to ensure even a minimal level of success would be to install draconian censorship measures. Still, it is not certain that the controls would be effective. Therefore, alternatives to control and censorship should be considered, such as developing increased suicide prevention activities on the Internet to counterbalance Internet suicide promotion activities. It is rare that persons involved in suicide prevention enter chat discussions to dissuade suicidal persons from killing themselves and encourage them to seek help. Also, public education over the Internet could be enhanced to facilitate ways and means to obtain help in the interest of suicide prevention.

References

Alao, A. O., Yolles, J. C., & Armenta, W. (1999). Cybersuicide: The Internet and suicide. *American Journal of Psychiatry, 156*(11), 1836–1837.

Australian IT (2004, August 4). Crackdown on suicide chat rooms. Retrieved from http://australianit.news.com.au/wireless/story/0,8256,10340811,00.html

Baume, P., Cantor, C. H., & Rolfe, A. (1997). Cybersuicide: The role of interactive suicide notes on the Internet. *Crisis, 18*(2), 73–79.

Becker, K., El-Faddagh, M., & Schmidt, M. H. (2004). Cybersuizid over Werther-Effekt online: Suizidchatrooms und-foren im Internet. *Kindheit und Entwicklung, 13*(1),14–25.

Becker, K., Mayer, M., Nagenborg, M., El-Faddagh, M., & Schmidt, M. H. (2004). Parasuicide Online: Can Suicide Websites Trigger Suicidal Behaviour in Predisposed Adolescents? *Nordic Journal of Psychiatry, 58*(2), 111–114.

Becker, K., & Schmidt, M. H. (2004). Letters to the editor: Internet chat rooms and suicide. *Journal of the American Academy of Child and Adolescent Psychiatry, 43*(3), 246.

Biddle, L., Gunnell, D., Owen-Smith, A., Potokar, J., Longson, D., Hawton, K., et al. (2012). Information sources used by the suicidal to inform choice of method. *Journal of Affective Disorders, 136*(3), 702–709.

Bonger, B. (2002). *The suicidal patient: Clinical and legal standards of care* (2nd ed.). Washington: American Psychological Association.

Booth, J. (2005, February 14). St Valentine's Day mass suicide pact fears. Times ONLINE, Retrieved from: http://www.timesonline.co.uk/article/0,,3–1484028,00. html

Braintech Inc. v. Kostivk (1999). 171 D.L.R. (4+h) 46, British Columbia, Canada

Bushman, B. J., & Anderson, C. A. (2001). Media violence and the American public. *American Psychologist, 56*(6–7), 477–489.

Calder v. Jones (1984). United States Supreme Court, 465 U.S. 783.

Commonwealth of Australia (2004b). House of Representatives Official Hansard, No 12, Wednesday, 4 August 2004, 30035–32038.

Commonwealth of Australia (2004c). House of Representatives Official Hansard, No 12, Wednesday, 11 August 2004, 32473–32480.

Criminal Code Amendment (Suicide Related Material Offenses) Act (2005). No. 92 assent 6 July.

Dobson, R. (1999). Internet sites may encourage suicide. *British Medical Journal, 319*, 337.

European Union (1999). *The European Union safer Internet plan.* EU-Decision Number 276–1999, Brussels: EU

Geist, M. (2002). *Internet law in Canada* (3rd ed.). Concord: Captus Press.

Harding, A. (2004, December 9). Japan's Internet "suicide clubs." BBC News. Retrieved from: http://news.bbc.co.uk/go/pr/fr/2/hi/programmes/ newsnight/4071805.stm

Hawton, K., & Williams, K. (2001). The connection between media and suicidal behaviour warrants serious attention. *Crisis, 22*(4), 137–140.

Innes, J.(2003, October 1). Coroner calls for police watch on web chat rooms, *The Scotsman*, Retrieved from: http://news.scotsman.com/topics. cfm?tid=746&id=1086122003>

Japon: Suicide collectif par Internet [Reuters]. (2004, October 13). *Le Devoir*, p. B6.

Luxton, D. D., June, J. D., & Fairall, J. M. (2012). Social media and suicide: A public health perspective. *American Journal of Public Health, 102*(S2), S195–S200.

Mehlum, L. (2000). The Internet, suicide, and suicide prevention. *Crisis, 21*(4), 186–188.

Mishara, B. L., & Weisstub, D. N. (2005). Ethical issues in suicide research. *International Journal of Law and Psychiatry, 28*, 23–41.

Niezen, R. (2013). Internet suicide: Communities of affirmation and the lethality of communication. *Transcultural Psychiatry, 50*(2), 303–322.

Pair planned suicide online police (2003, April 9). New Report RE; Europe. Retrieved from: http://iafrica.com/news/worldnews/227377.htm

Phillips, D. P. (1974). The influence of suggestion on suicide: Substantive and theoretical implications of the Werther Effect. *American Sociological Review, 39*, 340–354.

Pirkis, J., & Blood, R. W. (2001). Suicide and the media, *Crisis, 22*(4), 146–154.

Pirkis, J., Neal, L., Dare, A., Blood, R. W., & Studdert, D. (2009). Legal bans on pro-suicide web sites: An early retrospective from Australia. *Suicide and Life-Threatening Behavior, 39*(2), 190–191.

Polder-Verkiel, S. E. (2012). Online Responsibility: Bad Samaritanism and the influence of Internet mediation. *Science and Engineering Ethics, 18*(1), 117–141.

Rajagopal, S. (2004). Suicide pacts and the Internet: Complete strangers may make cyberspace pacts. [Electronic Version]. *British Medical Journal, 329*, 1298–1299. Retrieved 6 January 2005 from: http://www.bmj.com.

Reany, P. (2004, December 6). Internet pourrait encourager les suicides collectifs. *Le Devoir*, p. B6.

Richard, J., Werth, J. L., & Rogers, J. R. (2000). Rational and assisted suicidal communication on the Internet: A case example and discussion of ethical and practice issues. *Ethics and Behavior, 10*(3), 215–238.

Robertson, L., Skegg, K., Poore, M., Williams, S., & Taylor, B. (2012). An adolescent suicide cluster and the possible role of electronic communication technology. *Crisis, 33*(4), 239–245.

Seven die in suicide pacts, bringing death toll to 22 (2004, September 22). *New York Herald Tribune*, p. 3

Shepherd, J. (2004, March 6). Suicide blamed on chatrooms. *Birmingham Post.* Retrieved from:
http://icbirmingham.icnetwork.co.uk/0100news/0100localnews/tm_objectid=14 022277%26method=full%26siteid=50002-name_page.html

Smith, G.H., Bird, & Bird (2002). *Internet Law and Regulation* (3rd ed.). London, UK: Sweet & Maxwell.

Stack, S. (2000). Media impacts on suicide: A quantitative review of 293 findings. *Social Science Quarterly, 81*(4), 957–971.

Stack, S. (2003). Media coverage as a risk factor in suicide. *Journal of Epidemiology and Community Health, 57*, 238–240.

Stack, S. (2005). Suicide in the media: A quantitative review of studies based on nonfictional stories. *Suicide and Life-Threatening Behavior, 35*(2), 121–133.

Thompson, S. (1999). The Internet and its potential influence on suicide. *Psychiatric Bulletin, 23*, 449–451.

6

Mental Health Online: A Self-Report and E-Learning Program for Enhancing Recognition, Guidance and Referral of Suicidal Adolescents

Rezvan Ghoncheh, Carmen E. Vos, Hans M. Koot and Ad J. F. M. Kerkhof

Suicidal adolescents are underrepresented in mental health care (Cheung & Dewa, 2007), partly because young people commonly do not share their suicidal thoughts with their parents or other adults (Eskin, 2003; O'Donnell et al., 2003). Thus, their suicidality, including both suicidal behaviours and thoughts, (Bridge, Goldstein & Brent, 2006), is likely to remain undetected. This chapter reports on the development of the online suicide prevention program Mental Health Online. This program includes a self-report instrument to help adolescents recognize their suicidal thoughts and e-learning modules for training mental health gatekeepers to better identify and help suicidal adolescents. We then present the implementation of the program on the website http://www.MentalHealthOnline.nl.

Suicide and the Internet and the potential of online services

As of 2011, 94 per cent of the Dutch households have access to Internet, and 86 per cent of the Internet users go online daily or almost every day (Statistics Netherlands, 2012). Thus, the Internet is a powerful communication and information distribution tool in the Netherlands which can play an essential role in the promotion of mental health and prevention of mental health disorders. This is especially the case when it comes to youth suicide, which is surrounded by social stigma, taboo and high thresholds for help seeking. Several reasons highlight the value of Internet use in the case of adolescent suicide prevention: First, the simplicity and accessibility of the Internet makes it the first place adolescents and care providers turn for answers and information. Second, the Internet can be searched in private, making people feel at ease with topics they feel uncomfortable about. This is surely the case for a sensitive subject like suicidality that, when handled within the discretion and anonymity of the Internet, creates a low threshold of accessibility that is especially important for those adolescents that are looking for information and help. Third, the information offered can reach a very large audience with little effort due to the flexibility of the Internet. As a result, preventive efforts can be applied in various ways, addressing different target groups at the same time. As such, schools and mental health care institutions can easily be connected to create effective prevention programs. Finally, since the information can be procured casually to such a large audience, it can even have a taboo-breaking function. These advantages can reduce the high threshold for seeking professional help and the help-negation process for adolescents that struggle with suicidality.

Adolescent suicidality is a serious problem and needs vigilance and attention especially when considering that prior suicide attempt is one of the most important risk factors for suicide (Brent et al., 1999; Gould et al., 2003). That is why in 2009 a group of experts was assigned the task by the Dutch government to make an inventory of suicide prevention and intervention programs (De Groot, Kerkhof & De Ponti, 2009). This inventory highlighted, among many other things, the need for a Dutch validated self-report questionnaire that detects suicidal adolescents from various cultural backgrounds. However, prevention of suicidality requires more than a questionnaire. If suicidal adolescents are identified using a questionnaire, professionals who work directly with adolescents, also known as gatekeepers, should also be able to guide and refer them for treatment. Thus, the inventory also emphasized the need for tools to educate gatekeepers on the subject of suicidality. Based on the outcomes of the inventory, suicide prevention among adolescents has become one of the focuses of the Dutch House of Representatives since 2009. In 2011 the departments of Clinical- and Developmental psychology at VU University in Amsterdam started a government-funded program called Mental Health Online, which aims to stimulate suicide prevention among adolescents through online resources by developing an online self-report instrument to detect and referral those at high risk and online modules for gatekeepers focusing the identification, guidance and referral of suicidal adolescents.

Suicidal adolescents are more likely to disclose thoughts and feelings in self-report questionnaire than in face-to-face contact (Scott et al., 2009). Using a questionnaire thus enhances the possibility to identify and refer high-risk youth who would remain undetected otherwise (Scott et al., 2009). Moreover, it enhances the likelihood that high-risk youth actually receive treatment (Gould et al., 2009). However, the process of screening to promote early identification of high-risk youth often is inefficient, expensive and time consuming. The use of the Internet for the application of an online self-report instrument may solve these problems. First, online screening may save valuable time since the assessment can take place outside class or treatment. Second, since the self-report can be completed anywhere online, it will be easier to assess a large population including high-risk groups such as absent students or no-shows. In addition, participation can be enhanced by the dispatch of automatic reminders. Third, online screening is favourable because it allows youths to respond in their own place and time as they feel most comfortable, which makes the screening process less unpleasant for them. In addition, questions that are not applicable can be passed automatically, contributing to a personalized and shorter assessment. As a result, a broader population can be reached, and attrition may be limited. As a final point, because online screening allows the results of the assessment to be computed and forwarded directly, care professionals can react instantly in case of high risk. Thus, online screening is faster and safer than the general approach of paper and pencil assessment.

Since professionals who work with adolescents on a daily basis can play an important role in suicide prevention, the second part of the Mental Health Online program is aiming to enhance the process of recognition, guidance and referral of suicidal adolescents among this group. While Dutch gatekeepers are willing to contribute to suicide prevention, they are unfortunately not always successful in their efforts. The first, and probably the main, reason for this is that potential gatekeepers have the false impression that asking questions about suicidality to adolescents can actually make them become suicidal. This is why the subject of suicidality itself remains often unaddressed when engaging in a conversation with an adolescent they suspect to be suicidal. Second, gatekeepers often have little time to participate in training and courses to enhance knowledge on the subject due to their busy schedules. Often, the trainings and courses focusing on suicidality take at least one day, so these courses are not well adapted to the gatekeeper's schedule. These two obstacles combine to contribute to the fact that gatekeepers have little knowledge when it comes to suicidality, which in turn makes them quite insecure when interacting with suicidal adolescents. Educating gatekeepers through online resources could be a new approach for this problem. Gatekeepers can go online at any time to get access to training modules, also known as e-learning modules, that offer them basic information as well as skills and guidelines in prevention of adolescent suicidality. Furthermore, they can choose which e-learning modules they want to take depending on their own needs.

The suicide prevention program Mental Health Online has been developed in three stages. First, the proposed self-report is being validated using online assessments. Second, the effectiveness of the discussed e-learning modules is being investigated by carrying out an online randomized trial. Third, both parts of the program will be implemented using online resources. The development of the self-report started in 2009, and the development of the e-learning modules followed in 2011.The study protocol for Mental Health Online has been approved by the Medical Ethics Committee of the VU University Medical Centre Amsterdam. The next section provides a description of both aspects of the program separately and discusses how both aspects will be integrated during implementation.

Research Part 1: development of a self-report instrument

Objective

The first component of the Mental Health Online study is the development of a self-report instrument for assessing suicidality among adolescents age 12 to 20 from various cultural backgrounds. The instrument will be suitable for use in schools, youth health care, residential youth care, and on the Internet. This research will result in the availability of a tool that will meet the needs of health professionals, health care teams in high schools, general practitioners, youth care institutions, youth mental health care workers, public health departments and all caretakers who are likely to be in contact with suicidal youths.

Design

The study consists of three phases: (1) the item pool construction, (2) the pilot study in which the initial factor structure of the instrument will be determined within clinical and normal adolescent populations, and (3) the main study in which the predictive validity of the instrument will be determined within a normal multicultural population.

Instruments

The new self-report instrument is called the VOZZ, which stands for Questions on Suicide and Self-Harm (Vragen over Zelfdoding en Zelfbeschadiging). The questionnaire was developed to tap suicidal thoughts and behaviours as well suicide enhancing risk conditions, and include items on recent and past suicidal thoughts and behaviour, general and cultural risk factors and life events. Based upon the results of the projected study, the VOZZ will be shortened to become a quick and easy-to-administer self-report questionnaire. Questionnaires measuring suicide ideation (SIQ-JR) and depression (BDI-SF) are included during the study for validation and screening purposes.

Procedure

The VOZZ is administered online either in class or via a personalized link through e-mail and takes approximately 10 minutes to complete. A score on suicidal thoughts and depressive symptoms will automatically be computed and sent directly to the respondent by e-mail. In the case of a high score, the result will also be sent to the assigned care professional in the school, as well as a requests for a confidential talk with a care professional. The care professional then invites the concerning adolescents for a talk and assesses the need for eventual follow up and referral. The respondents are informed about this procedure before participation and again as they receive their results.

Research Part 2: development of e-learning modules

Objective

The second component of the Mental Health Online program is to enhance adolescent suicide prevention by training mental health gatekeepers through e-learning modules. This will be done by focusing on the process of recognition, guidance and referral of suicidal adolescents according to the model that underlies the QPR Gatekeeper Training, which is an internationally recognized program for suicide prevention and stands for Question, Persuade and Refer (Quinnett, 2007). According to this model, which was created by Paul Quinnett in 1995, the outcome of a suicide crisis will be better when three important steps are realized. First, early detection of warning signs associated with suicidality is an essential aspect of suicide prevention by gatekeepers. Second, gatekeepers should ask questions about the presence of suicidal thoughts, feelings and plans when having a conversation with someone who might be suicidal. By doing this, a conversation will start that can persuade the suicidal person to accept a referral for help, which is the third step of this model (Quinnett, 2007).

Participants

The main target groups in this study will be members of health care teams at schools, youth nurses and members of mental health services. However, other gatekeepers are allowed to participate in this study as well, but the study recruitment will primarily focus on these three groups.

Design

This study consists of two phases: first, a pilot/feasibility study which includes testing different aspects of the research process; second, the main study which will evaluate the effectiveness of the e-learning modules through a randomized controlled trial. Participants will obtain access to eight e-learning modules and will be tested three times, at baseline, immediately after attending the modules, and at a follow-up three months later. They will be tested on their level of knowledge regarding adolescent suicidality and also their perceived level of self-confidence in dealing with it. Both of these aspects will be tested using online questionnaires that have been developed for this study. Knowledge will be measured by asking questions about cases of adolescent suicidality, while self-confidence will be tested by questions and statements regarding the gatekeeper's perceived ability to interact with suicidal adolescents.

Instruments

The process of recognition, guidance and referral in the case of adolescent suicidality is addressed through eight modules (see Table 6.1), and each module captures different aspects of this process by educating, skill training, or offering guidelines to gatekeepers. The modules have been developed by the researchers in this study using Adobe Presenter 7 software to convert PowerPoint slides into e-learning modules. All modules are in Dutch.

The e-learning modules have several important characteristics and qualities. First, they are offered online and are accessible 24/7. Second, the content of the modules has been created in collaboration with experts on the subject of adolescent suicidality. Third, the modules are not time-consuming; each module takes only up to ten minutes. Fourth, the modules are easy to operate and have several attractive features such as graphs, cases, quizzes and voice-over. Finally, packages

Table 6.1   The eight e-learning modules of Mental Health Online program

Module	Aim
1. Suicidality among adolescents	Introduces the subject of adolescent suicidality
2. Risk factors	Reviews the risk factors which underlie adolescent suicidality
3. Ethnicity	Offers skill training when interacting with adolescents from ethnic minorities
4. Recognition of suicidality	Discusses how to recognize warning signs associated with suicidality
5. Conversation with the suicidal adolescent	Offers skill training on how to engage in a conversation with a suicidal adolescent
6. Conversation with the parents	Offers skill training on when to approach the parents and how to engage in a conversation with them
7. Suicide first-aid	Discusses the required steps when an adolescent attempts suicide
8. Care and aftercare (for schools)	Offers schools guidelines regarding the process of care and aftercare when students commit or attempt suicide

of the eight modules are defined for specific target groups according to the user's professional position and responsibilities. Users may identify with any target group and follow the selected modules or choose the full array. Furthermore, participants will also have access to additional information such as Dutch articles, films and interesting links on the subject of adolescent suicidality. An essential feature on the website is the online discussion board where participants can exchange thoughts with other gatekeepers on adolescent suicidality, and they will also have the opportunity to ask a group of experts questions regarding this subject. The modules and the additional information will be accessible for participants on the website http://www. MentalHealthOnline.nl.

Research Part 3: integration and implementation

Once the Dutch self-report has been validated (see Research Part 1) and the effectiveness of the e-learning modules has been investigated (see Research Part 2), a ninth module will be developed in which the self-report will be discussed. In this particular module, gatekeepers will find relevant information regarding the self-report instrument, such as how to score it and norms for the questionnaire, and at what score adolescents are considered at-risk for suicidality. This way, the self-report instrument can be used by the gatekeeper as an additional tool when engaging in a conversation with a possibly suicidal adolescent in order to obtain a more accurate perception of their level of depression and suicidality. By integrating the self-report instrument in the e-learning modules, gatekeepers will be provided a comprehensive online suicide prevention program that captures all the necessary steps and skills in the process of early recognition, guidance and referral of suicidal adolescents, which should also increase their level of confidence in helping suicidal adolescents.

It is expected that the program Mental Health Online will become available nationwide on the website http://www.MentalHealthOnline. nl as of 2014 for all the gatekeepers in the Netherlands. The program will be offered free of charge, giving the gatekeepers the opportunity to enrol in the program whenever they want from any given location, as long as they have access to the Internet. Depending on their prior knowledge and skills, gatekeepers can choose which e-learning modules are relevant for them to attend, creating a customized course for each participant. Gatekeepers can attend the e-learning modules at their own pace, and interrupt and resume the module at any given time, which is a valuable asset for those with busy schedules. Moreover, the e-learning modules can be attended as often as possible which gives the gatekeepers the opportunity to refresh their knowledge and skills whenever they want to. This way, the threshold to participate in an adolescent suicide prevention course will be reduced, and gatekeepers have an opportunity to help suicidal youths that otherwise might have remained unnoticed.

Another way to reach out to high-risk youths who would not be addressed otherwise is to make the self-report instrument available separately as a self-test on the Internet. Since youths commonly seek information and help anonymously online, the instrument can be used by youths who are not in school or in mental health care. After completion, an automatic advice will be sent based on the outcome of the self-test. Using this tool, suicidal youth may realize that they are in need of help, and subsequently they may make use of the offered (online) help. The instrument may also serve as an entry for online help such as chat services, and guided and unguided self-help courses to lead the users to the most suitable online and offline help available.

Conclusion

The program Mental Health Online is an online suicide prevention program designed for adolescents and their gatekeepers consisting of two components. First, eight e-learning modules will become available to gatekeepers which focus on the process of recognition, guidance and referral of suicidal adolescents. Second, a self-report questionnaire will be made available to detect suicidality among adolescents at an early stage. By offering the program online, participants can benefit from the advantages associated with Internet use over face-to-face training. First, the program will be available 24/7 from any location as long as the participant has Internet access. Second, applicants can complete the e-learning modules at their own pace and choose which modules are relevant for them, creating a customized training that meets the needs of each gatekeeper. Third, the package will be accessible for an unlimited number of participants simultaneously. Finally, this suicide prevention program will be offered free of charge since it was developed with limited effort and resources, and the maintenance of the two components will cost little. Additionally, the self-report will also be embedded in websites that promote mental health and suicide prevention, making the questionnaire more accessible for adolescents, and increasing the chances that at-risk youth can be appropriately referred and treated at an earlier stage of suicidality.

The idea behind Mental Health Online is that the suicide prevention program discussed in this chapter will be the first program in a series of prevention programs on mental health disorders that are going to be developed, investigated and offered online. When the effectiveness of these e-learning modules has been proven by research, e-learning modules can be developed for other important key issues. For instance, e-learning modules can be established to create awareness among members of the social network of people with a mental health disorder in order to build a more understanding environment. Furthermore, separate e-learning modules can also be established for parents, who can play an essential role in the recognition, guidance and referral of adolescents with mental health disorders or those who are facing problematic life circumstances. Lastly, awareness and help-seeking behaviour could be improved through e-learning modules educating those with mental health disorder(s). By addressing all the important key figures, programs on prevention and intervention of mental health disorders will be more effective.

The opportunities provided by the Internet also facilitate the connection between prevention and intervention programs, and research, which is essential in the development of effective programs. Internet use creates a safe study environment, limiting any ethical concerns regarding potential emotional effects and burden on vulnerable populations, since participants can be assessed online and monitored directly by the researchers or involved caretakers. In cases of acute risk, they can react immediately. People will also be more willing to participate in research programs since the required effort and commitment on their part will be limited when using the Internet for data collection. Moreover, data will be saved automatically and can be analyzed directly without the trouble of collecting them in person and manually importing them. Furthermore, Internet use also allows one to monitor fluctuations in mental health and well-being, and to promote mental health in the long term. Finally, the online element makes it possible to reach and train key figures that can simultaneously play an important role in prevention of mental health disorders.

Today, the Internet is the first place people turn when facing uncertainties. It allows people to stay in their own comfort zone while gaining knowledge on topics that are surrounded with social stigma and taboos. It is therefore important that people have access online to accurate information and tools in searching for solutions for their problems. Online programs can guide and encourage people to take the required steps toward facing their problems which can only be achieved, especially when it comes to adolescents, by reducing the threshold to find help through awareness and education. Mental Health Online aims to accomplish this by serving as a portal for online prevention and intervention programs on mental health disorders.

References

Brent, D. A., Baugher, M., Bridge, J., Chen, T., & Chiappetta, L. (1999). Age- and sex-related risk factors for adolescent suicide. *Journal of the American Academy of Child & Adolescent Psychiatry, 38*(12), 1497–1505. doi: 10.1097/00004583–199912000–00010

Bridge, J. A., Goldstein, T. R., & Brent, D. A. (2006). Adolescent suicide and suicidal behavior. *Journal of Child Psychology and Psychiatry, 47*(3–4), 372–394. doi: 10.1111/j.1469–7610.2006.01615.x

Cheung, A. H., & Dewa, C. S. (2007). Mental health service use among adolescents and young adults with major depressive disorder and suicidality. *Canadian Journal of Psychiatry, 52*(4), 228–232. Retrieved from http://publications.cpa-apc.org/media.php?mid=355

De Groot, M., Kerkhof, A. J. F. M., & De Ponti, K. (2009). Onderzoek naar aspecten van suïcide in Nederland 2008–2012: Een quick scan. Retrieved from GGZ Nederland website: http://www.ggznederland.nl/kwaliteit-van-zorg/suicidepreventie/quick-scan-definitief.pdf

Eskin, M. (2003). A cross-cultural investigation of the communication of suicidal intent in Swedish and Turkish adolescents. *Scandinavian Journal of Psychology, 44*(1), 1–6. doi: 10.1111/1467–9450.t01–1–00314

Gould, M. S., Greenberg, T., Velting, D. M., & Shaffer, D. (2003). Youth suicide risk and preventive interventions: A review of the past 10 years. *Journal of the American Academy of Child & Adolescent Psychiatry, 42*(4), 286–405. doi: 10.1097/01.CHI.0000046821.95464.CF

Gould, M. S., Marrocco, F. A., Hoagwood, K., Kleinman, M. Amakawa, L., & Altschuler, E. (2009). Service use by at-risk youth after school-based suicide screening. *Journal of the American Academy of Child & Adolescent Psychiatry, 48*(12), 1193–1201. doi:10.1097/CHI.0b013e3181bef6d5

O'Donnell, L., Stueve, A., Wardlaw, D., & O'Donnell, C. (2003). Adolescent suicidality and adult support: The reach for health study of urban youth authors. *American Journal of Health Behavior, 27*(6), 633–644. doi: 10.5993/AJHB.27.6.6

Quinnett, P. (2007). QPR gatekeeper training for suicide prevention: The model, rationale and theory. Retrieved from http://www.qprinstitute.com/pdfs/QPR%20Theory%20Paper.pdf

Scott, M. A., Wilcox, H. C., Schonfeld, I. S., Davies, M., Hicks, R. C., Turner, J. B., & Shaffer, D. (2009). School-based screening to identify at-risk students not already known to school professionals: The Columbia suicide screen. *American Journal of Public Health, 99*(2), 334–339. doi: 10.2105/AJPH.2007.127928

Statistics Netherlands (2012). Statline. Retrieved from http://statline.cbs.nl/statweb/?LA=en

7
Avatars and the Prevention of Suicide among Adolescents

Xavier Pommereau

This chapter describes the development and use of digital avatars in the prevention of suicide with teenagers and young adults. Twenty years ago, in November 1992, we created the first hospital unit in France specifically dedicated to caring for suicidal adolescents and young adults (Pommereau et al., 1994). Located downtown in a satellite building of the Centre Hospitalier Universitaire de Bordeaux, this unit and two others (a child psychiatry unit for pre-adolescents and a unit for anorexic and bulimic youths) form the Pôle Aquitain de l'Adolescent, which also includes a department for outpatient consultation. This 15-bed "suicidology" unit is an open institution that cares for suicidal adolescents brought in by emergency and intensive care services as a back-up to psychiatric care (80 per cent of the patients admitted), and young people admitted as a preventative measure following repeated serious behaviours that we consider suicidal, even if the person committing these acts does not recognize them as such (alcoholic comas, running away and threatening suicide, intentional reckless driving, unprotected or non-consensual sex, etc.). Stays are deliberately brief, around three weeks, and the multidisciplinary team of psychiatrists, psychologists, nurses and social workers has three objectives: (a) conduct a thorough medical-psychological assessment of the young patient, bringing in family members and speaking with them; (b) work on expressing emotions and suffering, both in one-on-one and group sessions; and (c) improve acceptance of psychiatric care so that this patient group, known for disregarding follow-up recommendations, becomes more cooperative with later outpatient care. Approximately three hundred patients stay with us each year, with a total of 350 visits (some patients are admitted two or three times). While methodological biases certainly exist, several follow-up surveys showed a substantial reduction in repeat attempts and severity of their somatic condition among patients admitted in the year following their admission (Pommereau et al., 1995).

In our twenty years of experience, we have seen the patients we admit grow younger (the average age decreasing from 17 to 15), and the types of behavioural issues associated with suicide have changed; in particular, we have seen a drop in panic attacks and a considerable increase in three types of issues: binge drinking leading to alcoholic comas, bulimic episodes followed by provoked vomiting, and self-harm such as scarification, burns and abrasions (Pommereau, Brun & Moutte, 2009). Like intentionally suicidal actions, these self-injurious behaviours expose two intents – the first conscious, and the second much less so: (a) to let go of their suffering, to forget it, get it off their chest; and (b) to show their despair to the world, with the secret expectation that they will be seen, recognized and helped (Pommereau, 2005, 2006 and 2011). Without knowing it, these adolescents attempt to escape their suffering, while at the same time revealing their pain to those around them, with an insistence and repetition that show an irrepressible need to feel that they exist. And these young people do so with captivating, upsetting images, at levels proportionate with their needs.

To understand this development, remember that society has been profoundly affected by the digital revolution, as has adolescence. Today's adolescents are children of the audiovisual era: they are "photographed" in their mother's womb (high-resolution 3D ultrasounds), captured from every angle in pictures and videos from birth onward, force-fed material and symbolic consumer goods from a young age (food "rich" in proteins, fats and sugars; TV and video game images; interactive toys and stuffed animals, etc.), and are permanently connected to consoles, music players and screens. From an increasingly younger age, these digital natives know how to "project themselves" more through images than words. I call them "teens. com" because their lives are posted online, sometimes more than they know, through their images, posturing, showy gestures, pictures and Facebook profiles. They show who they are, what movements and trends they belong to, what they like and don't like, who they have ties with, etc. Teens who are doing well act out to a lesser degree: they cultivate their image, "brand" themselves with commercial goods or body modifications (piercing, tattoos), look for rites of passage, etc., but stick to moderate, aesthetic changes, to please themselves or to show off to their peers. However, teens who are not doing well go too far, expose themselves to dangerous situations, with the secret hope that we will find them and come to their aid. They express the breaks, cracks and wounds in their souls through excess – from "splits" to complete breaks – in the literal and figurative sense. These splits largely take the form of repeated relational "clashes," running away, truancy, drinking or abusing drugs, self-harm, Internet and computer addictions that cut them off from the real world, problematic eating behaviours, abortions from unwanted pregnancies, etc. These teens literally cut into their flesh, into their relations with other people; they exaggerate the marks and signs they wear to "cut" themselves away from their peers, to be recognized with a new identity, one that is negative. This is not a matter of pleasure, but a need to escape misery and suffering any way possible. And to not be alone, maybe to form a "group of bodies" that is even more visible and identifiable; they link themselves to other troubled youth. As the saying goes, "birds of a feather flock together" – teens search for belonging, relationships that will smooth over the cracks in their psyche.

We were convinced that these teens have a lot to express by posting themselves from different angles, though they said very little in interviews. We then decided to change our care practices. Our goal was to facilitate expression in all forms, respecting the integrity of the subject, that is to say, the other and its relationships with other people, while authorizing a release of some violence – though it remains contained, permissible, showcased in a non-damaging context. This allows the subject to better "read" his state of being by taking a step back, gaining some distance. Thus our patients gradually become capable of seeing their difficulties and are therefore able to understand them in order to better cope with them. Why let these teens, once again stuck with "nothing to say," emphasize these shortcomings? Why not make use of their resources – often substantial but left unused? We believe that it is always better to support someone's skills if we want to help them in a lasting fashion, so we created new therapeutic workshops with them, based on self-representation. And, to play with words, you could say that we wanted to bring ourselves into the age of the avatar – the embodiment of the self, whose etymology comes from the Sanskrit avatāra, meaning "incarnation, descendant of Vishnou on Earth". Before deciding to use digital avatars, we explored more traditional forms of self-portraits, with our directions to teens being to "show yourself and your suffering, through forms and images". We were surprised by the success of our experiment: no teens refused to draw or paint themselves "and their suffering".

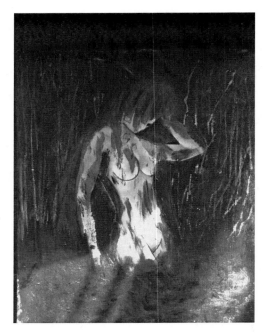

Figure 7.1 "Through Fire and Blood" self-portrait by Clara, 16, Abadie Centre (author's private collection)

We also realized that – even though they were open to using pens, markers, coloured pencils and paint – they especially appreciated being able to represent themselves using a stuffed animal or something that belonged to them (often a souvenir from early childhood) that they then modified to illustrate their suffering. How? Often, they would amputate a limb; this was the case for Jessica, 16, a teenager who had been raped when she was eight years old. She represented herself using this one-legged doll with black tears flowing from her eyes and marks from the criminal hands of her abusive cousin on its body, as well as the self-inflicted burns and scarification that this sexual violence triggered.

The most recalcitrant teens, those most "blocked" from putting their suffering into words, turned out to be the most engaged in these forms of representation. On the other hand, it must be said that using materials strongly associated with childhood proved important, as if these patients were trying to match their past to their current identity-based

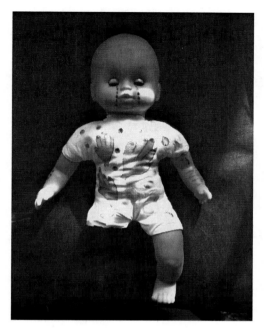

Figure 7.2 "Self-portrait", Jessica, 16, altered doll, Abadie Centre (author's private collection)

tensions. And behold, these sullen teens.com, scarred and with a look out of Dante's Inferno, gave caretakers their works "to hold onto," mostly saying they were "OK" if they had to follow further instructions. Since we wanted patients to get hands-on, and because reminders of their childhood were necessary at this stage, we asked them to create figurines of themselves out of modelling clay. The idea didn't surprise them – some of them were astonished that we hadn't thought of sculpting as a medium for self-expression earlier. All of the teens welcomed this new approach.

This is how Jordan, 15, a "black with an Afro that all the girls love" according to the other patients, was able to "create" himself, although he couldn't manage to join "the top and the bottom" of his figure. He was "really sorry" about it, he said. He would have liked "for the whole thing to hold together". He didn't realize yet how he had just expressed a part of his story through this image. Jordan is an adopted child. What does he know about where he came from? Practically

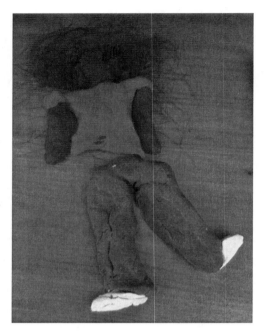

Figure 7.3 Artwork by Jordan, 15, figurine made of modelling clay, Abadie Centre (author's private collection)

nothing, other than that he was left in a Haitian orphanage from birth until he was three years old. Over time, he convinced himself that his biological parents were so poor that they had decided to save their son by leaving him with nuns. As for his adoptive parents, Jordan loves them wholeheartedly, "he owes them everything, he knows that," but they seem unable to understand him, they are always too quick or too flexible, inconsistent – as if following educational principles they never grasped the basics of, or even the point. "They adopted me because they couldn't have children," Jordan specifies, admitting that he "acts like a tyrant towards them to make them react". He knows that, which only keeps him from acting correctly. He would like to howl in distress, but who would be able to recognize him, without judging him? So he doesn't say a word. But doesn't the apparently coincidental break in his effigy represent the successive heartbreaks he could have experienced, from birth, even conception, until his abandonment in unknown circumstances? And isn't the fact that he is

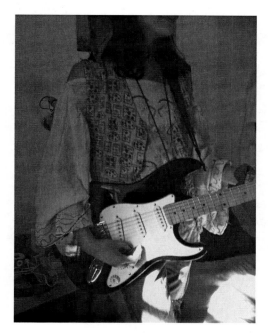

Figure 7.4   "Guitar Hero back from everything", form by Léa, 14, Abadie Centre (author's private collection)

torn between his two "histories" what makes him suffer so? We won't ask him the question now, given the state he is in – less than fifteen days after attempting to hang himself – we won't imply that he is that appalling figure whose body is separated at the waist.

Figurines made of modelling clay and images created through looks and postures: there is only a small step from playing to personifying, expressing distress and dreams, openly sharing their wants and skills, then relaxing their bodies, thoughts and roles.

In 2011, we were ready to start with digital avatars, using the rich graphical palette provided by The Sims software: Over the course of one individual session with a staff member, in front of a computer and with the chance to view oneself in a physical looking-glass attached to the screen, each patient had to produce their digital double, dress it and give it accessories, as realistically and as close to their appearance as possible. This projection exercise was a huge success, offering some support to the

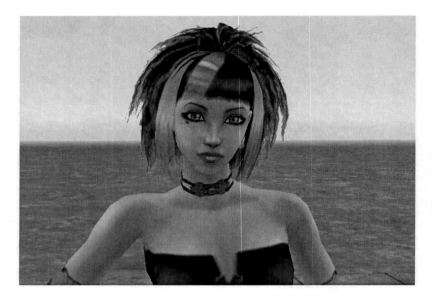

Figure 7.5   Avatar for Sandra, 14, Centre Abadie (author's private collection)

healer-patient relationship with teens whose digital culture allows them to say with images what they had trouble saying otherwise. And we were able to observe that this projective ego-concentration encouraged verbalization and dialogue, prompting teens, absorbed by the choice of features and attire available, to talk about themselves, their similarities and differences compared to loved ones, and to reflect on their place in their family, as well as their expectations and fears.

Because of this very elaborate dialogue opener from a large software producer, we are now creating a serious game, one that places patients' avatars in situations known to be critical (family tension, school bullying, breakups and emotional losses, etc.). This program, currently in development, will be available in 2013 and focuses less on animation and graphical rendering of characters (much less meticulous than in the Sims) than it does on the detailed conversation trees possible between avatars and non-player characters. The objective will be to help each patient better grasp the more sensitive aspects of his or her tension points, with the help of a caregiver. How does he behave when faced with this difficult situation? Why does she react the way she does? What could he have done to have a more balanced attitude? Why is that impossible for him now? Briefly put, it will be a new form of mediation, a support to patient-caregiver relationships, a psycho-dynamic application of virtual reality therapy (VRT) techniques, inspired by exposure methods used in cognitive behaviour therapy. These techniques have been used for over a decade as a therapeutic tool in psychiatry, with the basic principle being to immerse patients in controlled virtual environments that have been specifically designed for the issue to be treated. First developed for the treatment of phobia, their use will undoubtedly become more and more common for some suicide prevention teams.

This presentation of our therapeutic journey is intended to show that treating suicidal teens and young adults can no longer rely on traditional individual and group sessions. Lacking adequate words to relate their pain, they need support, mediation that facilitates expressing their emotions.

Note: The photographs used in this chapter have been kindly provided by the author. They are his exclusive property. Use of these photos, in whole or in part, outside of this document is subject to copyright rules.

References

Pommereau, X. (2005). *L'adolescent suicidaire* (3rd éd.). Paris: Dunod.

Pommereau, X. (2006). Figurabilités corporelles à l'adolescence. Des conduites d'agir aux actes de soins en institution. *Adolescence, 24*(3), 623–639.

Pommereau, X. (2011). *Nos ados.com en images. Comment les soigner.* Paris: Odile Jacob.

Pommereau, X., et al. (1994). La prise en charge des jeunes suicidants. *Revue Soins, Psychiatrie, 169.*

Pommereau, X., Brun M., & Moutte, J.-Ph. (2009). *L'adolescence scarifiée,* Paris: L'Harmattan.

Pommereau, X., Delorme, M., Tedo, P., Druot, J. M., Caule-Ducler, E., & Hernandez, D. (1995). Pourquoi hospitaliser les adolescents suicidants ? In F. Ladame, J. Ottino, & C. Pawlak (eds), *Adolescence et suicide* (pp. 185–191). Paris: Masson, coll. Médecine et Psychothérapie.

8
Crisis Chat: Providing Chat-Based Emotional Support

Mary Drexler

Crisis Chat (accessible at www.crisischat.org) is a program of CONTACT USA, a national membership-based organization whose membership includes over 50 crisis centres in 20 states across the country. Until 2010 its mission had been to provide leadership and support to centres that provide helpline services to people in crisis or need. In 2010, one of CONTACT USA's centres, CONTACT Lifeline, a program of Family and Children's Service of the Capital Region in Albany, NY, brought the concept of online emotional support via chat services to the attention of our national organization as a means to reach out to underrepresented populations who may not be comfortable with talking with someone over the telephone.

The rationale behind online chat services is substantiated by research indicating 79 per cent of all adults within the United States are on the Internet and 93 per cent of all teenagers, 12 to 17 years of age, are on the Internet (Pew Research Center, Internet and American Life Project, 2013). People in distress are reaching out online more and more. Online communication is more convenient, allows anonymity, is a means for reducing stigma and shame and often a means for testing the water to see if there is someone who really cares and is willing to listen. The majority of Crisis Chat users (about 70 per cent) are under the age of twenty-five.

From the start, we realized that although online emotional support through chat services had some common denominators with help by telephone, it most certainly had some major differences. Chat relies only on text communication. Audible cues are lost, so staff and volunteers must frequently ask questions for clarification of what has been said. Another difference is that the average length of chats is forty-five minutes to one hour, with a high-risk chat taking two hours or

96

longer. Although some calls may be that same length, chats are consistently longer in length. Chats tend to be longer due to the slower form of communication; it takes longer to type than to speak, and there also tends to be a high level of disclosure paired with higher-risk situations.

CONTACT USA's goals for Crisis Chat were as follows: to provide people with tools to make better health/life decisions, to increase culturally relevant access for support for current and emerging generations, and to decrease stigma associated with accessing mental health and other support services. Online emotional support via Crisis Chat is not counselling or therapy; it is compassionate, non-judgmental listening, an exploration of thoughts and feelings, suicide risk assessment, and a definite exploration of positive next steps and options. In provision of services through Crisis Chat we refer to the individual requesting services as the chat "Visitor" and the staff/volunteer providing the emotional support as the chat "Specialist," an individual specially trained in crisis intervention, suicide prevention and intervention, and online communication.

So what is the key to providing effective online emotional support? In our first two years of experience providing Crisis Chat, we learned many lessons about what key elements are necessary to provide online emotional support. First, at the beginning of each chat we learned it is important to inform the Visitor about the purpose of chat. The Specialists inform the Visitors that we are there to discuss their issues and provide them options that can support them during their difficult times. We inform them that chat sessions are generally 45–60 minutes in length, which helps them focus on their immediate concerns. Specialists are aware though that chats may take longer depending on the Visitor's level of distress.

Second, the Specialist needs to be assertive in the chat process and at times remind the Visitor that they need to focus on the critical issue of the moment, allowing the Specialist to better support them and provide appropriate options to handle their crisis. Third, and very important, it is essential that the Specialist be patient and allow for conversation to flow. Chat is a slower medium of communication, and the Visitor needs to be allowed to tell their story.

We found that in order to be successful from the start of a chat, gathering as much information from the Visitor upfront in a brief survey has proven to be extremely helpful. Although a Visitor can choose to remain anonymous to some degree, there are a few questions required to be answered prior to entering chat, including:

- Age
- Zip Code
- What are you concerned about today? (select one)

1. *Suicide*	8. *Physical and/or emotional abuse*
2. *Depression*	9. *Bullying*
3. *Anxiety*	10. *Eating disorder*
4. *Relationship issues*	11. *Self-harm*
5. *Family issues*	12. *Sexuality issues*
6. *Financial issues*	13. *Physical health*
7. *Addictions*	14. *Other:*

- How upset are you today? [Scale of 1–5]

1. = *I'm doing OK*	4. = *Very upset*
2. = *A little upset*	5. = *Extremely upset*
3. = *Moderately upset*	

These questions are found to be essential in focusing the Visitor and in helping the Specialist identify the primary distressing issue and current emotional state of the Visitor.

Other crucial issues to keep in mind as a Specialist are: the online disinhibition effect, the potential for out-of-sync communication, the lack of auditory cues, and the need for "checking in." First, online disclosure is usually higher than disclosure on telephone helplines. Chat Visitors may not always answer the Specialist's questions as they are too busy typing out more and more details regarding their current problems. This practice by the Visitor requires the Specialist to be more assertive than they might be if they were handling a crisis phone call. Questions will often need to be repeated to help the Visitor focus on one issue at a time.

Second, out-of-sync communication is not uncommon in chat environments. For Visitors who don't chat online much, this occurrence may create confusion. It is the role of the Specialist to clarify which Visitor answer is a response to which Specialist question and vice versa so as to avoid undue confusion. Third, without auditory cues, communication can certainly become more challenging. The Specialist needs to clarify the meaning and emotion connected to the chat content. Fourth, more than usual checking-in may be required on some chats, as auditory cues are not obvious. One cannot hear if someone may be crying, or angry, etc. Appropriate questions to ask include:

- "How are you doing with this chat? Are you still okay?"
- "How are you feeling right now? Any changes we should talk about?"
- "Am I hearing you right? Do you feel we are on the same page"

As mentioned earlier, about 70 per cent of our chats are from individuals under twenty-five years of age. This population often finds it difficult to engage in conversation, written or verbally, that focus on coping strategies, safety planning or connections with community resources. The result of this hesitation often leads to challenges in communication online. Some of these challenges presented by teens or young adults include:

- The use of one word or short answers especially when the Specialist initiates safety planning or next steps conversation.
- The common use of "I don't know" ("idk") by the teen or young adult.
- The lack of insight about their feelings and difficulties in visualizing any solutions that might work for them.

To deal with these challenges the Specialist must spend time rephrasing, being persistent, and being creative with their approach with the young Visitor; a question such as "What advice would you give a friend in this situation?" might be helpful in moving forward. Also, although it is tempting as a Specialist to come with a plan or solution for young Visitors, the focus should be on empowering the young person. A happy medium that can help is to have them come up with their own solutions and provide general helpful suggestions, such as reaching out for help, expressing their feelings in writing, etc.

Safety planning is especially difficult with young Visitors as they may be experiencing high levels of distress and are having trouble thinking proactively. Significant trauma issues or physical or emotional health issues might also create barriers for engaging in safety planning. In these cases it is essential that the Specialist accept the limitations of the Visitor, balancing that with assessment of immediate safety. The Specialist needs to be sensitive to the fact that the Visitor may not be ready to move forward with formal help. One thing we have learned in Crisis Chat is that safety planning is often completed only partially, if at all, in some cases.

As Crisis Chat welcomes Visitors experiencing a vast array of emotional crises, it is our practice to ensure each Visitor is currently safe and not at imminent risk due to their current emotional and or physical circumstances. During each chat, we ask the Visitor if they are currently having suicide ideation or thoughts of suicide and if they had had any of these in the past. If the answer is yes, the Specialist must complete a suicide assessment. An example of a question that can begin this conversation is:

- "You seem to be experiencing so much stress right now – have you been thinking of suicide?"

If the Visitor is uncomfortable with answering the question when first asked, the Specialist can come back to the question at a later time in the chat after the Visitor has shared more about their current circumstances. As chats can sometimes come to an abrupt end, it is often helpful to ask the suicide question early in the chat conversation. The full risk assessment can be completed later in the chat. We have found that when asked about suicide, approximately 42 per cent of Visitors indicate they are thinking of suicide at the time of the chat. Based on this percentage, there is a good chance there may be frequent situations where risk can be high and potentially imminent. In these instances, it becomes imperative that the Specialist attempt to collect location and contact information from the Visitor. If a Visitor is not open to giving consent for rescue and is not willing to provide information on their location, there is still a possibility they can be found using their Internet Protocol (IP) address (available through some chat software programs). The following are steps a Specialist can follow to send rescue to a Visitor that has refused to provide other, more direct, contact information:

1. Run the IP address through an online IP address location finder: i.e. www.whatismyipaddress.com to see if it correlates to the zip code provided during registration (pre-chat survey completed by the Visitor). This will also provide information on the Internet Service Provider (ISP) which is for that particular IP address.
2. Once the ISP is determined, you can use the ISP legal department look-up tool at www.search.org/programs/hightech/isp/ .
3. Call law enforcement for the Visitor's zip code and give them that IP address, the ISP and its legal department's contact information, the Visitor's risk level, and any other identifying information you may have.

Despite this process for locating someone at imminent risk for suicide, there are several limitations. While IP addresses are sometimes helpful, they are often not as reliable as say phone numbers collected via caller ID systems. An IP address is attached to a computer and may not provide real information on the Visitor's actual physical location. Even if a location can be determined, it may be part of a larger physical location such as a university, apartment complex, or Wi-Fi network. Another challenge is that law enforcement may not always be willing or able to take the extra steps to contact and work with an ISP to locate the Visitor. It is thus up to the Specialist to be persistent and to follow-up to ensure a connection was made and an effort is being made to locate the Visitor at risk. The process of locating someone who is chatting online can take several hours to unfold, and rescue may not be possible. In reality, as with taking crisis calls, taking online chats relies heavily on the Specialist's ability to listen, care, and build a positive working relationship with the Visitor so that taking more intrusive measures, like contacting law enforcement, can be avoided.

There is a certain etiquette that the Specialist should be trained to understand. It is essential to create an environment where both the Specialist and the Visitor feel comfortable and safe. Proper etiquette includes:

- Answer a request for chat as promptly as possible.
- Respond promptly to messages and expect the same from Visitors.
- Use correct punctuation and minimize spelling errors; do not use slang in conversations; maintain professionalism (use emoticons sparingly).
- Refrain from joking with Visitors. There is a greater chance for miscommunication in the absence of verbal tone.
- Do not type in all CAPITALS as this is translated as "shouting" and is considered rude in online communication.

For new Specialists, there are several common issues with which they may struggle. For some, not knowing how to fill the silences that may occur can be difficult. It is essential in moments of silence to use validating and empathetic statements summarizing what the Visitor has been conveying and to also type minimal encouragers that may be used when handling a crisis call. These include "mmmm," "hmmmm," "really," etc. For others, not knowing when to respond or how long a response should be can create a challenge. When providing help online, short chat segments work best, as it takes a bit longer to write than talk. It is important to also match the Visitor's style as much as possible, however, remaining professional at the same time. Another concern for some Specialists is that it is difficult to know if they are being successful in connecting with the Visitor. One must remember it may take longer to develop a sense of rapport as the luxury of tone of voice is not present. Finally, as the Specialist first embarks on providing online help, there is a tendency to want to move too quickly to problem solving or a suicide risk assessment with the Visitor because they don't know where else to go early on in the chat. However, just like on phone crisis work, it is important to use open-ended questions, validation, and empathy at the beginning of chat as a means for allowing the Visitor to express their issues that brought them to chat in the first place.

Ending chats may also be difficult. There are some definite do's and don'ts related to ending a chat. The Do's include:

- "How are you feeling now compared to the beginning of the chat?"
- "I am going to be wrapping up the chat in 5–10 minutes so let's summarize where you are at now and what plans we have discussed for moving forward."
- "Before ending the chat, I would also like to provide you with the national helpline number should you wish to connect with someone and chat is not available when you need it."
- "Thanks once again for using chat services. Please come back if you find yourself in need of support or resources to get through a difficult time."

The Don'ts include:

- "I have to go now."
- "Sorry, I have to take a call. Come back later."
- "We have been chatting quite a while; I think it's time to end the chat."
- "We don't have any more time to chat now. I have someone else waiting to chat."

There is one last note about chat endings. We have learned in our experience providing chat services that there will be times when a Visitor will abruptly end the chat. It is easier online than on a phone call for a Visitor to disconnect as there is less of a feeling of responsibility to the relationship. It is easier to leave someone you can't see or hear. The frustration with this type of disconnect is that we often have no way of "calling back" Visitors who have not provided contact information.

As an organization considering the development of chat, you will find that there are a variety of issues/challenges that you may encounter.

CONTACT USA's crisischat.org has received chats on some of the following (keep in mind many of the Visitors have been under 25 years of age): financial concerns; mental health concerns; self-harm behaviours; bullying-related issues; eating disorders; LGBTQ issues (Lesbian, Gay, Bi, Transgender, Questioning); and suicidal ideation, thoughts, and attempts, etc. The following are sample chat scenarios and strategies for addressing some of these issues raised:

Scenario

You have been on a chat with a man who is severely depressed, has not left his apartment in one week, has law school debt of $150,000 and has no job and doesn't like his chosen career, doesn't see his children much, thinks he is a terrible father, and thinks everyone (including himself) would be better off if he were dead. You have been chatting with him for two hours. He has not de-escalated his wish to die (but has no plan or means or time set) and he also seems very intent on continuing the conversation with you.

Response

- Acknowledge that he is dealing with multiple stressors and recognize how much strength it took for him to reach out to share this with someone.
- Review with him identified buffers/supports.
- Develop and/or review his safety plan if his thoughts of suicide increase or become more severe (i.e. plans, means, intent).
- Encourage him to prioritize the challenges he is facing, perhaps focusing on one thing rather than all of it at the same time (more manageable steps).
- Provide him with phone numbers (for local hotline and crisis centres, national hotlines like the Lifeline's 800–273-TALK(8255) in the U.S., and local resource directory services like 2–1–1 in the U.S.), so he can talk more with other service providers if needed and also ask for information about local free or low cost counseling services.
- Remind him he can return to Crisis Chat in the future.

Scenario

You have been on a chat with a Visitor who states she was raped two days ago and also has a history of childhood sexual abuse; she just can't take the pain anymore and she wants to kill herself. She seems to be in great pain, but she is taking an average of 2–3 minutes to respond to you each time you respond to her. It is still early in the chat interaction, with discussion focusing on the Visitor's reasons for dying and the difficult emotional content she's brought to chat.

Response

- Acknowledge that what she is going through sounds intense and commend her for being so brave to reach out for help.
- Express concern for her in light of the topics she has brought to chat.
- Remind her you are here to listen to her if she is ready to engage in chat.
- Ask her about her current safety and physical status (is she in need of medical care?).
- Don't push her to file a police report if she is has expressed she doesn't want to do this; advise that there are resources (e.g. RAINN in the U.S.) that can help explain details around physical exam, reporting, and different state laws.
- Address her desire to kill herself. Ask about desire, intent, capability/means.
- If long pauses continue, ask clarifying questions to see if she is so overwhelmed with emotion that she's having difficulty typing/replying. If she is multi-tasking, gently ask her if she can focus just on the chat and that this will help you provide her with as much support as possible.
- If she cannot focus just on chat, encourage her to come back, and before she leaves chat provide her with phone numbers and websites to access for more support and information.

Scenario

You are chatting with a 15-year-old girl who has disclosed that she has an incurable disease that will affect her for the rest of her life. It makes her smaller than other girls and she walks with a limp. She seems to be very distressed, and when you begin your suicide risk assessment, she says she wants to die, but seems to ignore your other questions regarding previous attempts and past thoughts of suicidality. She has a lot to say and is expressing her anger and hopelessness to you.

Response

- Give her space to vent – it's good that she is able to express the emotions she is experiencing (she may even answer some assessment questions without you even having to ask them).
- Look for possible buffers and supports and continue to remain alert to possible warning signs that her suicide risk is high.
- Provide occasional cues that you are reading/listening so that she knows you are still there (e.g. "hmmm," "ok," and "I see").
- When there's a break in her messages OR if her venting seems more destructive than productive, jump in with short messages to get her attention.
- Ask her very concise/direct questions that do not re-open the door to long venting.
- Remind her you are very interested in what is causing her distress and that you have some questions that will facilitate further discussion.
- Things to keep in mind when chatting with a teenager:
- What may not seem like a big deal to you may seem very serious to them.
- Don't talk down to them or attempt to "be the adult."
- Encourage them to talk with family, but don't push this too much, especially they're already expressed fear, anger, or distrust.
- With this case, keep in mind that depression often accompanies physical conditions/ailments. Ask questions that will help you detect signs of sadness, hopelessness, and helplessness.

Scenario

A woman is chatting with you about her husband who has been missing for five days, she suspects on a drug binge. She says she is worried for his life and worried about providing food for her children in his absence.

Response

- You need to explicitly ask how the Visitor is feeling, how she is coping.
- Because you cannot hear the tone of her voice, she might be angry, have no affect, or she may be crying hysterically. You just don't know unless you ask.

- You should ask questions that further explain "worried" – what does that mean exactly? Get her to describe what this means to her.

Scenario

You are chatting with a young woman who tried to kill herself two months ago with pills but survived and never told anyone. She has disclosed for the very first time on chat that she thinks about suicide frequently and she is afraid for her life. You start to encourage her to reach out to an adult in her life, but she says she won't tell anyone. You talk to her about positive coping strategies, but she says nothing works.

Response

- It was perhaps too early in the chat to start encouraging her to reach out to an adult in her life – she JUST reached out to chat. Talk with her a little bit and find out what it is she's going through.
- Ask her how frequently she is thinking of suicide (worrying / rumination).

Scenario

You are chatting with a teenage girl who is being bullied in school because she is a lesbian. She has no friends and she feels very alone. You ask her if she is thinking about suicide today, and she says yes, and then she talks about all the reasons she has for not wanting to go on anymore.

Response

There are three main issues at play here: suicidality, bullying, and potential issues around her sexual orientation.

Suicidality

- Let her continue to chat, emote about her reasons to die, and when you are able, later on, continue the assessment (past history, means, intent, etc.).
- Engage in safety planning.

Bullying

- Tell her bullying is unacceptable and NOT her fault.

- Encourage her to speak to a trusted adult and not to keep her feelings inside (telling someone may help her feel less alone).
- Talk about how to stand up to kids who bully. If speaking up seems too hard or not safe, encourage her to walk away and stay away, and to not fight back.
- Talk about strategies for staying safe, such as staying near adults or groups of other teens.
- Encourage her to do what she loves: special activities, interests, and hobbies can help boost her confidence.

Sexual orientation (if a concern to her)

- Let her know she is not alone, you are here to listen.
- If she would like, offer her contact info to a national support service (like the Trevor Project in the U.S.) that specializes in engaging with LGBTQ youth.

Scenario

You have been chatting with a teenage girl who is resisting the urge to cut as she doesn't feel pretty or wanted; her boyfriend broke up with her last week. You have asked her if she can put the razor down while she is talking to you when she says she has to go and leaves the chat.

Response

- At this point, there is nothing more you can do for the Visitor.
- For the Specialist (from a supervisor's perspective): remind the Specialist that abrupt endings are common on chat and that the Visitor may have obtained what she needed ... someone to just listen to her concerns and to let her know there are people in the world who care about her well-being.
- Supervisor: review the chat transcript in order to give the Specialist constructive feedback.

Scenario

You are chatting with a man who has not slept in three days and has had suicidal ideation, but is not at immediate risk. You have been chatting for 90 minutes, and as you try to move him towards safety planning, he gives you many one word answers, and you feel as if you are carrying the conversation.

Response

- Ask a check-in question, like: "How are you doing now that we've been chatting for a while?" ... "What are you thinking about?" "How are you feeling?"
- Depending on his response, you can then lead into more planning questions, like:
- "Based on our conversation so far, what are some things you'd like to try to stay safe?
- "You've expressed to me that you've had some thoughts about suicide – what are some things you can do if those thoughts come back or become more serious?"

[Note: the above questions are open-ended, inviting the Visitor to elaborate more.]

[If needed, remind the Visitor that we are here to listen and help him consider his options and develop a safety plan. We are not here to tell him what he should or should not do.]

Providing chat services to Visitors in crisis can be an intense experience, especially in high-risk situations. Additional challenges that can be expected include:

- Visitors telling you too much information or constantly repeating themselves;
- Visitors presenting with multiple issues and unable to focus;
- Visitors that seem helpless in identifying internal and external coping mechanisms (especially youth); and
- Visitor reluctance to reach out for further help (declining more long-term resources offered).

Despite these challenges, the Specialist's role remains the same as with other emotional support and crisis services. As with crisis phone work, the Specialist needs to demonstrate a willingness to gain a clear understanding of the issues presented by each Visitor, validate how the Visitor is feeling and build a rapport with them that will increase the chances they will be more willing to explore other resources by the end of the chat. Empowering the Visitor should be a primary goal for the Specialist. The Specialist should not try to convince the Visitor of what they need to do, but trust that the Visitor can help him/herself with the Specialist's support.

For those we connect with through online communication the results have been quite positive and Visitors' responses to Crisis Chat have been positive:

- "I have gotten a lot of support here. I would go as far as to say they have saved my life."
- "This service has been a great help to me. It is a great alternative when you can't or don't feel comfortable talking on a phone. I know I've tried to call the suicide hotline three times, but panicked each time, so this is perfect for me."
- "Being in my current situation I have no support, it was nice to have or feel as though someone was on my side."
- "I was really relieved to see this service existed cause I hate talking on the phone."
- "I think this is an incredible service and resource for those of us who are suffering and just need someone to listen to us."

Clearly, there is a need for emotional support provided via a chat environment. CONTACT USA has learned since the launch of Crisis Chat in 2010 that despite its challenges, chat, text, tweeting and other technologies are the only way to reach out to underserved populations, specifically the generations who have grown up in today's technology age.

Many thanks to the following, some of whom provided assistance during the development of Crisis Chat and others that continue to support the Crisis Chat program by providing the actual chat service:

Agora Crisis Center, Albuquerque, New Mexico
Arkansas Crisis Center, Springdale, Arkansas
Austin Travis County Integral Care, Austin, Texas
Baton Rouge Crisis Intervention Center, Baton Rouge, Louisiana
Centerstone, Nashville, Tennessee
Community Crisis Services, Inc., Hyattsville, Maryland
ContactLifeline, Inc., Wilmington, Delaware
CONTACT Lifeline, a program of Family and Children's Services of the
   Capital Region, Albany, New York
CONTACT of Mercer County, Ewing, New Jersey
CONTACT The Crisis Line, Jackson, Mississippi
Crisis Center of Johnson County, Iowa City, Iowa
Crisis Clinic, Seattle, Washington
Grassroots Crisis Intervention Center, Inc., Columbia, Maryland

Life Crisis Center, Salisbury, Maryland
Mental Health Association of Frederick County, Frederick, Maryland
Mental Health Association of Montgomery County, Rockville, Maryland
National Suicide Prevention Lifeline (Now known as "Lifeline")
Samaritans Inc., Boston, Massachusetts
Samaritans, UK
The Support Network, Edmonton, Alberta (Canada)
The Trevor Project
eMental Health, Canada

References

Pew Research Center, Internet and Amercian Life Project (2013) Accessed 12 May 2013 http://www.pewinternet.org/Static-Pages/Data-Tools/Get-the-Latest-Statistics.aspx

9

The National Suicide Prevention Lifeline and New Technologies in Suicide Prevention: Crisis Chat and Social Media Initiatives

Gillian Murphy

The National Suicide Prevention Lifeline (Lifeline), 1–800–273-TALK (8255), is a free and confidential service for those in emotional distress or suicidal crisis. In calling the Lifeline, individuals across the United States who need immediate assistance are connected to the nearest available crisis centre within a national network of more than 160 centres. The Lifeline is funded through the US Substance Abuse and Mental Health Services Administration (SAMHSA) and partners with the National Association of State Mental Health Program Directors (NASMHPD) and with Living Works, Inc., an internationally respected organization specializing in suicide intervention skills training. Established in 2005, the Lifeline has answered over three million calls and currently responds to over one million calls a year.

Crisis hotlines and suicide prevention

The Lifeline network centres provide a unique and accessible resource to the community in general and to individuals at risk of suicide in particular. Often underutilized by the mental health community, these crisis hotlines can provide low-cost access to professionals and/or paraprofessional volunteers that are specifically trained in suicide assessment and intervention. Available 24 hours a day, crisis centre staff can take the time to thoroughly evaluate a caller's suicidal ideation, provide support and guidance, offer referral information, develop a safety plan, and if needed dispatch emergency intervention to the scene. While network centres are independently owned and operated, they must adhere to standards of service related to suicide risk assessment and follow imminent risk guidelines established by the Lifeline. These evidence-informed standards and guidelines reflect the Lifeline value of taking all action necessary to prevent an individual from dying by suicide, and the Lifeline pursuit of innovative and effective practice includes a concerted focus on cultivating the preventive and supportive capacity of new media in suicide prevention.

In the United States, more than 37,000 people die each year by suicide (Centers for Disease Control and Prevention (CDC), 2012). Many of these are people that were previously seen in the emergency department (ED) or inpatient setting. Unfortunately, following discharge, as many as 70 per cent of suicide attempters never attend their first appointment or maintain treatment for more than a few sessions (Appleby et al., 1999; Boyer et al., 2000; Tondo, Albert & Baldessarini, 2006). Individuals are discharged to a system that is fragmented, fraught with service gaps and significantly underfunded: a system that lacks the care coordination that is critical in the period following admission to an ED or inpatient setting. The need to establish a formal "chain of care" for those at greatest risk is evident, and services that are flexible and multifaceted can be more responsive to the needs of the community than a focus on traditional service provision alone (Pirkola et al., 2009). In fact, a recent report by the Clinical Care Intervention Task Force (a working group of the National Action Alliance for Suicide Prevention – a public-private partnership with the goal of advancing the U.S. National Strategy) identified five elements critical for public and behavioural health organizations to adopt in order to effectively address suicide prevention in their communities. One of these elements focuses on the significant importance of providing immediate access to care for those at risk for suicide. It calls for 24/7 services to be available to those in crisis and, in particular, mentions the benefits of having crisis lines and online crisis chat/intervention services available in order to reduce barriers related to "cost, distance, and stigma" – factors that can significantly impede access to care (Covington & Hogan, 2011). The provision of online and telephonic care, available 24/7, convenient, with a high degree of anonymity, and at low to no cost for those seeking care is essential in order to facilitate access to help during times of crisis.

Lifeline use of chat and text-based services

The increasing use of chat and text services can be seen from new media usage reviews. According to the Pew Internet & American Life Project's

Mobile Access 2012 report, 72 per cent of cell phone users reported using their cell phones to send or receive text messages (compared to 65 per cent in May 2009) (Smith, 2012). This increase is not isolated to youth, as may be expected. Over 60 per cent of 45 year olds were found to be just as likely to use SMS as they were to make voice calls from their mobile device. In fact, text messaging and chat are gaining on email as the preferred means of daily communication.

The availability of a text or chat service to those in crisis may facilitate reaching out for help by those reluctant (or unable) to call. Research suggests that individuals may be more willing to reveal sensitive information about their thoughts, behaviours and values through electronic means than in person (Bryant et al., 2006). Two well-known suicide prevention organizations have demonstrated significant success in their implementation of chat and text services to their crisis hotline networks. The Samaritans UK, following a successful pilot, began providing emotional support via text messaging service at Samaritans' 201 branches throughout the UK and Republic of Ireland. From the start of the pilot in April 2006 to the end of 2007, Samaritans received over 258,000 text messages from people experiencing feelings of emotional distress and despair, and this was achieved with no active publicity of the text message number (www.samaritans.org). In addition, The Lowdown, a New Zealand-based initiative that serves to address depression in young people, provides text, chat and email services that can be accessed from their website (www.thelowdown.co.nz). A recent evaluation of their service showed that young people's response to the use of this service was extremely positive and service use was higher than expected. For example, in the six months from June to December 2008, 58,517 texts and 1,817 emails were received and sent. The number of unique users of the text service doubled during this time. In addition to this, requests for online assistance from the Lifeline more than tripled over 2011. From October to December 2011, the Lifeline received 111 suicidal comments to the Lifeline Facebook page, over 1500 direct requests from Facebook to assist users, and 105 emails from people asking for help who did not want to talk on the phone.

While the Lifeline contracts with a national crisis centre to provide email responses to online requests for help, this process is not optimal. Email cannot provide the immediate response that those in crisis likely need. Few of the many outreach emails result in ongoing communication with the individual in crisis, despite the often urgent request for online assistance. For some the crisis may have passed, but for others the situation may have worsened and the need for Lifeline to expand the capacity for crisis centres to respond to users online and in real time is critical; for many individuals, text and chat services are the only means of communication they will use. Over the past few years, centres within the Lifeline network have begun to expand service provision to offer chat- and text-based services locally. For the Lifeline, the task has involved harnessing this expertise into the creation of one national network where individuals across the US could access chat services at any time through one portal.

The first element that influenced the Lifeline development of chat services was the participation in a chat program made available for veterans. In 2007, the Veterans Crisis Line was established through a partnership between the Lifeline and the US Department of Veterans Affairs. Callers to the Lifeline are given the option to "press 1" if they are a veteran, family member, or active duty member of the military, and calls are routed to the Veterans Crisis Line (www.veteranscrisis-line.net) in Canandaigua, NY. Since its launch in 2007, the Veterans Crisis Line has answered more than 600,000 calls and made more than 21,000 potentially life-saving rescues, and the call volume continues to rise. By 2009, the Veterans Crisis line was also seeing an increased number of requests for online assistance – particularly from active duty veterans abroad, and a decision was made to add an online chat component. Named the Veterans Chat program, this service has since helped more than 50,000 people, with numbers growing daily. A unique aspect of the Veterans Chat program is the availability of a "self-check quiz" for veterans to complete prior to entering the chat system. This quiz, adapted from the Interactive Screening Program developed by the American Foundation for Suicide Prevention (www.afsp.org), is an anonymous web-based screening tool that begins with a brief assessment of stress and depression. Items related to Post Traumatic Stress Disorder (PTSD) and Traumatic Brain Injury (TBI) have been added for use with veterans. Visitors to the web page can choose to fill in this self-check quiz and, once submitted, will receive a reference code and a personalized written response from a crisis counsellor through the website within 30 minutes. Veterans are urged to enter the chat system to discuss their responses or can return to the chat system at a later date and supply the reference code, which allows the crisis counsellor to refer back to the previously answered quiz. The use of the self-check quiz has proved beneficial for both the crisis counsellor and veterans – it allows the veterans to spend some time in self-reflection, keeps them engaged should the chat service be temporarily busy, and provides the crisis counsellor with a means to engage the veteran right from the start by addressing their responses in various areas. Specifically, it allows for immediate assessment of the users' potential risk for suicide. Since its inception, the volume of chats received has increased rapidly from 23 a day in 2010, to 50 a day in 2011, and 106 per day in the first six months of 2012. Individuals that enter this system that are not associated with the US military are transferred to one of two designated back-up centres within the Lifeline network. In 2012, a texting option was added to this site – 838277 (VETALK) – this system has also shown tremendous growth in volume in the short time since its launch.

Another element that facilitated the Lifeline development of chat services was the participation of many Lifeline centres in the newly established "CrisisChat.org" program that had been launched under the guidance and direction of CONTACT USA (CUSA) (www.contact-usa. org). CUSA, a leader in the field of crisis line accreditation, is one of the few programs in the US devoted to establishing and maintaining standards of service at crisis lines, warm-lines, and reassurance calling programs. CUSA is the only accrediting agency that has developed standards for the provision of chat services within a crisis hotline setting. Their CrisisChat.org service began in 2010 with three crisis centres and, with minimal advertising, the chat service has steadily grown from only a few chats per day to up to 60 chats per day in 2012. As chat volume grew, CUSA added more crisis centres, providing them with technical support, clinical training and a website platform.

The Lifeline chat pilot was launched 1 March 2012. All chats entered the Lifeline network through one central portal located on the Lifeline home page (www.suicidepreventionlifeline.org). Although ultimately the preference would have been to route all incoming chats to the closest crisis centre, for the pilot, chats were routed to the next available centre and not by geographic location. Centres in the network accepted chats from any location within the U.S., while chats that originated outside of the U.S. were not permitted to enter the system. Those users were automatically referred to the International Association for Suicide Prevention (www.iasp.info) where a list of international crisis centres could be found. Each of the eighteen participating centres provided a minimum of four hours continuous coverage per day, and shifts for various centres were staggered across coverage hours Monday–Friday 5pm–1am. Crisis centres were expected to take two chats at a time per staff member. No particular software was required for participation in the pilot; however, all centres used either Sightmax (www.sightmax.com) or iCarol (www. icarol.com) chat software.

For the pilot, the Lifeline collected a limited amount of data. Much of the information was filled out by the user before entering the chat session. When the user entered the system, a brief pre-chat survey was presented which required that they provide their name/alias, age and gender. In addition they were asked the following: What is your main concern? (list of issues), Do you have thoughts of suicide? (Yes – Current, Yes – Recent Past, No) and How upset are you? (scale of 1–5). Upon leaving the session, the user was once again asked: Now that you have finished your chat session, how upset are you? (scale of 1–5) and, finally, was asked to provide general feedback on their experience. This post-chat survey was voluntary, and roughly 20 per cent of users complete this information. In addition to collecting data from the user, the Lifeline required that centres submit information on whether suicidal ideation was present, whether the user was at imminent risk for suicide, and whether attempts were made to dispatch emergency rescue.

During the nine months of the pilot (March 2012–September 2012), almost 17,000 individuals attempted to obtain support through the chat portal. Findings from a sample of 6,477 users indicated that chat participants were primarily female (74 per cent) and young, with 51 per cent being under the age of 19 and 83 per cent under the age of twenty-nine. The acuity level of the chats tended to be high with 58 per cent reporting being "very" or "extremely" upset upon entering the chat session and 59 per cent reporting "current" suicidal ideation. A total of 1,296 users completed both the pre- and post-chat surveys: Of 701 users that stated they were "very" or "extremely" upset upon entering the chat system, 62 per cent (433) reported an improvement in their mood by the end of the chat session. More general findings indicated that chat interactions took longer than typical calls. Although the average length of chats taken over this time period was 29 minutes, many chats took much longer with some running between one and two hours. Reports indicated that even though users tended to reveal sensitive information early on in the chat session, engagement, assessment, and intervention could take an extended period of time. Demand for assistance during the pilot far exceeded the ability of the crisis centres to provide services. While almost 17,000 individuals attempted to enter the chat system, roughly one-third of those did not result in an established chat session primarily due to extended wait times to connect to an available chat specialist. Chat operations were resource intensive, and due to the high intensity and high acuity level of chats, it was difficult for chat specialists to maintain four-hour shifts. The range of issues raised and the intensity of the interactions proved overwhelming over an extended period. Chat specialists did report that the pre-chat survey was helpful in focusing the chat session, as suicidal ideation could be immediately addressed, providing efficient use of available time.

A key issue that has emerged in the provision of chat services is the challenge that arises in locating an individual that is deemed to be at significant risk for suicide. The use of "active rescue" is standard practice for all Lifeline centres (active rescue referring to the need to initiate rescue with or without the caller's consent once imminent risk has been established), and though such rescue can be very difficult, it is not impossible. It is important to consider that while some centres have expressed reluctance to embark on online service provision for this reason, the difficulty that arises in locating an individual at risk is no longer particularly linked to the online world – the degree to which online services mimic phone services is increasing rapidly as individuals more and more rely on mobile phones and VOIP services as they call in to crisis hotlines – with both systems very difficult to trace. As part of the Lifeline recommendations to centres, we encourage each centre to build a relationship with their local law enforcement and Public Safety Answering Point (PSAP or 911 call centre) to inform them of their service and the difficulties presented. Centres must be sure to record the IP address and time stamp of the chat visitor. This information should be easily available to staff, who can then use it to find the City/State and Internet Service Provider (ISP) of the individual at risk (sites such as www.whatismyipaddress.com can be helpful). Whereas in the past, the IP address alone may have been sufficient to narrow down the location of a specific user, current IP sharing practices significantly limit the use of IP alone. Once the City/State is located, the associated zip code can assist in finding the local police department who should be provided with information that clearly indicates the risk of suicide and inability of the crisis centre staff to locate the user. Centres should request that the police contact the legal department of the ISP for information specific to the user. The ISP does not require a subpoena to give out private information to law enforcement when there is potential danger. They do, however, need to be clearly presented with the information related to risk and the specific time that the chat session was initiated. Again, while isolating the actual user can be difficult, it is not always impossible, and anecdotal reports have indicated that, once the PSAP has agreed to try to contact the ISP, crisis centres have experienced a high degree of success in locating the individual.

Despite challenges raised, the chat pilot was viewed as a successful and necessary service for those at risk of suicide. In 2013, the Lifeline formally launched Lifeline Crisis Chat. A formal partnership with CONTACT USA facilitated the addition of the CrisisChat.org centres and the establishment of a single national network of crisis centres with online crisis intervention expertise.

While the Lifeline focused initial efforts on chat-based services, there are several centres within the network that engage in text-based service provision. These programs tend to particularly target youth – such as the New York City-based Be Brave against Bullying initiative (www.uft. org/campaigns/be-brave-against-bullying) and the Nevada-, Texas- and Mississippi-based "text for teens" programs, which outreach to local schools in an effort to reach youth in crisis. In addition, in 2010 the Lifeline began to pilot a text message follow-up service with four Lifeline centres that reached out via text to individuals that had called the crisis line and were assessed to be at significant risk. Callers consented to receive follow-up contacts from the crisis centre and "opted in" to receive these contacts via text messages to further assess their status over the following few days or weeks. While the program proved helpful for callers, limited funding prevented the program from becoming more firmly established in crisis centre operations. The Lifeline plans to reassess the benefit of texting for both incoming contacts and follow-up services over the coming year. One model for follow-up of particular interest is an automated interactive text-messaging program recently piloted with veterans. Veterans received an automated text that asked them to rate their level of crisis on a numeric scale. If the individual responded at or beyond a designated threshold, an alert was sent to the provider, so they could follow-up by phone. Findings from this pilot are yet to be published (G. Rimaldi, personal communication, June 2011).

Lifeline and social media

According to the Pew Internet & American Life Project, 89 per cent of Internet users between the ages 18–29 (a high-risk population for suicide attempts) and 72 per cent of all online adults belong to social networking sites (Brenner, 2013) while 59 per cent of US adults look online for health information (Fox, 2011). The rapid development of social media has impacted how we think about suicide prevention in many ways: People use social media to communicate their thoughts of suicide, they leave virtual suicide notes to a mass audience, and they create memorial pages that can, if not monitored, lead to suicide contagion. People also use social media to educate, raise awareness and, most significantly, to reach out for help. On 11 November 2011, for example,

Ashley Billasano of Houston, TX sent 144 tweets to her followers asking for help, before completing suicide. On 5 January 2012, Jordon DuBois, a soldier stationed in Colorado, posted a suicide note to Facebook an hour before he died by suicide in a car accident. On 11 January 2012 Sinead O'Conner tweeted that she was unwell and in danger. She also used Twitter as a "cry for help" in September 2011. When you think about the fact that the average American has 634 ties in their social network (Hampton et al., 2011), when a suicide happens, a large circle of people are now witness to the event.

The Lifeline is actively involved in social media and online marketing for suicide prevention. In 2008, with the help of partners SPAN USA and Active Minds, the Lifeline launched the Lifeline Gallery (www.lifeline-gallery.org) with the goals of raising awareness about the effects of suicide, reducing stigma, connecting people to emotional support, and offering help. The Lifeline Gallery provided a safe space for survivors of suicide, suicide attempt survivors, those who struggled with suicidal thoughts, and those in the suicide prevention field to share their stories of hope and recovery. Users could choose a character to create an online representation of themselves (or avatar) and then use this character to share their story. Over 800 individuals shared their struggles with thoughts of suicide and stories of loss. While the Lifeline Gallery received an overwhelmingly positive response, as years passed traffic to the site declined substantially. In 2012, the Lifeline replaced this with a new video gallery on YouTube (www.youtube.com/800273TALK). The "My Lifeline" Video Gallery features personal stories from people who have called the Lifeline in the hope that these brief videos will inspire others to call when they are in crisis. The Lifeline also features videos from suicide prevention advocates, suicide attempt survivors, and suicide loss survivors.

The Lifeline works with the safety teams of all major social networking platforms to ensure there are procedures in place to assist any individual expressing suicidal ideation and/or intent. Facebook is one of the largest social networking sites today and, as such, has played a central role in the Lifeline efforts to address suicide prevention in online communities. In 2006, the Lifeline began a partnership with Facebook that focused on identifying an effective means whereby individuals who were concerned for someone at risk for suicide could report their concerns and offer assistance. Users that posted any suicidal comment or content that evoked concern for safety could now be flagged and reported to the Facebook safety team using the Report Suicidal Content link that was established (see www.facebook.com/help/contact/?id=305410456169423). Lifeline staff guided the approach of the Facebook safety team as they responded to users in crisis: The safety team provided support, encouraging the user to contact the Lifeline (1–800–273-TALK (8255), and then engaged the assistance of the Lifeline in reaching out to the user via email. In 2011, as part of a continued effort to reach people at risk, the Lifeline extended its partnership to offer crisis services via chat to people who had been reported for posting suicidal content. Now, when someone on Facebook is reported, the Facebook Safety Team reviews the report and, if appropriate, sends the at-risk user an email encouraging them to call the Lifeline 1–800–273-TALK (8255) or to click on a link to begin a confidential chat session with a crisis worker. Two centres within the Lifeline network are available 24 hours a day, seven days a week, to respond to Facebook users opting to use the chat system. This new service led to a surge of Lifeline Facebook fans. Since June 2011, the Lifeline has gained almost 25,000 additional "likes," bringing the total number to 48,549 (www.facebook.com/800273TALK).

In addition to the use of new media in suicide prevention, the Lifeline also focuses attention on approaches to online postvention. Social media significantly impacts what happens following a suicide and necessitates a change in postvention strategies. When someone dies by suicide, that person's social media profiles often become hubs for friends and family to talk about the suicide and memorialize the person who died. Exposure to suicide, whether through a personal connection or through the media, is an established risk factor for suicide. There is substantial evidence that certain messages (e.g., those that glamorize the suicide) and certain information (e.g., details regarding the method of suicide used) may contribute to contagion (see http://reportingonsuicide.org for more information). The comments posted on these profiles can contain unsafe messages and sometimes include expressions of suicidal ideation by friends or family of the deceased. Postvention strategies are particularly important when the deceased is between the ages of 15 and 24, as data indicates this age group is particularly active online and those most affected are likely already engaging in online conversation about the suicide. Accessing social media sites, therefore, provides an important and efficient means of distributing information and resources, as well as of monitoring those connected to the bereaved for any indications of suicide risk. The Lifeline recommendations on how to approach online suicide postvention efforts as well as how to safely memorialize someone who has died by suicide (including recommended language for website comments) can be found here: www.sprc.org/sites/sprc.org/files/library/LifelineOnlinePostventionManual.pdf.

The most recent suicide prevention strategy to be undertaken by the Lifeline, launched in the summer of 2012, is an online youth campaign, You Matter, which aims to persuade young adults in crisis to contact (call or chat) the Lifeline through the use of a microsite and social media (www.youmatter.suicidepreventionlifeline.org). Using social media alone as its promotional mechanism, You Matter will maintain two social media channels – Facebook (www.facebook.com/youmatterlifeline) and Tumblr (http://youmatterlifeline.tumblr.com) – in addition to existing Lifeline Twitter and YouTube channels to disseminate campaign content as appropriate. The You Matter campaign is evidence of the ways in which new media can influence approaches to suicide prevention and awareness. The hope is that You Matter will be spread and promoted by the target audience themselves to their social media friends and followers. In this way, You Matter uses social media as a way to move beyond informing young adults about the Lifeline and focus more on engaging them to join the conversation and, in turn, build awareness and trust. You Matter doesn't hide the problem of emotional distress or suicidal crisis; rather it speaks about these issues in a nonclinical manner. It doesn't highlight the word "suicide" and describes crises using linguistic imagery. Overall, the messaging is conversational and positive, providing a sense of hopefulness, and focuses heavily on spreading the positive message of "you matter." You Matter doesn't focus on the problem, but on the solution – that suicide is preventable with help.

For the Lifeline, the use of new media has become an essential component in all service delivery. The programs highlighted here reflect but a few of the ways in which online crisis intervention can serve to engage individuals at risk of suicide, enhance suicide prevention efforts, and positively impact the role that crisis centres play within the current mental health system.

References

Appleby, L., Shaw, J., Amos, T., McDonnell, R., Harris, C., McCann, K., … Parsons, R. (1999). Suicide within 12 months of contact with mental health services: National clinical survey. *British Medical Journal, 318*, 1235–1239.

Boyer, C. A., McAlpine, D. D., Pottick, K. J., & Olfson, M. (2000). Identifying risk factors and key strategies in linkage to outpatient psychiatric care. *American Journal of Psychiatry, 157*, 1592–1598. doi: 10.1176/appi.ajp.157.10.1592

Brenner, J. (2013). *Pew Internet: Social networking* (full detail). Retrieved 21 August 2013, from Pew Internet & American Life Project http://pewinternet.org/Commentary/2012/March/Pew-Internet-Social-Networking-full-detail.aspx

Bryant, J. A., Sanders-Jackson, A., & Smallwood, A. M. K. (2006). IMing, text messaging, and adolescent social networks. *Journal of Computer-Mediated Communication, 11,* 10–11.

Centers for Disease Control and Prevention (CDC) (2012). Deaths: Preliminary Data for 2010. Retrieved 8 March 2012, from http://www.cdc.gov/nchs/data/nvsr/nvsr60/nvsr60_04.pdf

Covington, D., & Hogan, M. (2011). *Suicide care in systems framework.* Washington, DC: National Action Alliance: Clinical Care and Intervention Taskforce.

Fox, S. (2011). *The social life of health information,* 2011. Retrieved 14 July 2012, from Pew Internet & American Life Project http://pewinternet.org/~/media//Files/Reports/2011/PIP_Social_Life_of_Health_Info.pdf

Hampton, K. N., Sessions Goulet, L., Rainie, L., & Purcell, K. (2011). *Social networking sites and our lives.* Retrieved 14 July 2012, from Pew Internet & American Life Project http://www.pewinternet.org/~/media//Files/Reports/2011/PIP%20-%20Social%20networking%20sites%20and%20our%20lives.pdf

Pirkola, S., Sund, R., Sailas, E., & Wahlbeck, K. (2009). Community mental-health services and suicide rate in Finland: A nationwide small-area analysis. *The Lancet, 373,* 147–153.

Smith, A. (2012). *Cell Internet use 2012.* Retrieved 14 July 2012, from Pew Internet & American Life Project http://pewinternet.org/~/media//Files/Reports/2012/PIP_Cell_Phone_Internet_Access.pdf

Tondo, L., Albert, M. J., & Baldessarini, R. J. (2006). Suicide rates in relation to health care access in the United States: An ecological study. *Journal of Clinical Psychiatry, 67,* 517–523.

10

Results and Experiences of 113Online, a Comprehensive Dutch Online Suicide Prevention Platform

Jan. K. Mokkenstorm, Annemiek Huisman, Ad J. F. M. Kerkhof and Jan H. Smit

The emergence of new information and communication technologies has led to the development of Internet based "e-mental health" interventions including e-therapy, online screening, tele-consultation and online information and education services. These developments can benefit the field of suicide prevention by increasing the availability, accessibility, and acceptability of care to suicidal individuals, being often emotionally vulnerable and ambivalent help seekers (McGinty et al., 2006; Krysinska & de Leo, 2007; Sarchiapone et al., 2009; Lester, 2008; Luxton et al., 2011; Barak, 2007). This chapter presents the Dutch online suicide prevention platform which provides several complementary services over the Internet. We first present the general background, introducing the potential contribution of e-mental health for suicide prevention. We then describe the organization of 113Online, the principles and key services they provide. Third, we present data on the characteristics of 113Online service users and their usage, as well as some outcomes, using data recorded during the first three years of operation. The final section summarizes and discusses our experiences to date and research findings. Plans for future developments will be presented and a research agenda will be proposed.

Background

Availability, accessibility, and acceptability of services are key issues in suicide prevention. A recent survey among 286 general practitioners in Great Britain indicates that a large majority of GPs view the availability of mental health services as inadequate, sometimes to a point that they refrain from referring at all to avoid disappointment of their patients (Saini et al., 2010). Other studies have established the dissatisfaction of patients who did receive specialist mental health care (Hengeveld et al., 1988; Pirkis et al., 2001; Taylor et al., 2009). These studies report that patients often experience a lack of respect and empathy, with professionals challenging their autonomy and declining them involvement in treatment decisions. The effect of this dissatisfaction on future help seeking is illustrated by Gould et al. (2012), who found that a third of callers to US crisis hotlines report a lack of trust or negative experiences as their reason for not accessing mental health care after their call.

Recent studies (Pagura et al., 2009, Bruffaerts et al., 2011; Gould et al., 2012) demonstrate that a high proportion of suicidal individuals receive no treatment. They found this to be only partly due to financial or structural barriers, such as the availability of services. Even in the Netherlands, a country with a well-established mental health system, 40 per cent of suicide attempters do not use mental health care services in the year preceding their suicide attempt, and 33 per cent had never used mental health services in their lives (Ten Have et al., 2011). As these studies show, suicidal individuals' attitudes towards help and help seeking appear to be main barriers.

Pitman and Osborn (2011) argue that the apparent rejection of mainstream (specialist) services by suicidal individuals calls for investment in settings and services that are more acceptable to them and satisfy their personal needs and preferences to a greater extent. Suicide prevention thus not only faces the challenge to increase availability of services, but also to increase their acceptability and effective use. This should involve the provision of self-care or informal care opportunities for those who prefer to work problems out by themselves, or living in regions with limited availability of health care services.

Internet-based e-mental health services can play a crucial role in meeting these challenges. The widespread use of the Internet in society allows for large-scale dissemination of education, self-help and therapy (McGinty et al., 2006). With large target audiences looking for useful information, empathy and validation on the Internet (Baker & Fortune, 2008; Harris et al., 2009), suicide prevention has an excellent opportunity to reach them with interventions and to counteract suicide propagating websites which also present themselves to suicidal Internet surfers (Durkee et al., 2011; Biddle et al, 2012; Gunnell et al., 2012).

Apart from logistic and targeting advantages, the privacy, anonymity and practicality of the Internet result in greater access to services. Individuals who hesitate to seek help because of shame, the wish to stay in control, or the fear to be disappointed or rejected, may enter (as well as leave) interventions with greater ease. A single click suffices. The physical distance to an online professional safeguards a great deal of autonomy and control that many patients find lacking or fear losing when seeking help in regular care. Seen in this light, online services may constitute an alternative or supplement gateway to effective mental health care for suicidal people that would otherwise not seek help and for patients that are dissatisfied with or inhibited in discussing suicidality with their therapist in ongoing regular treatment.

Research has shown promising results of different online interventions aimed at anxiety disorders, mood disorders and substance abuse (Spek et al., 2007; Andrews et al., 2010; Cuijpers et al., 2008). In the field of suicide prevention, however, there is a dearth of outcome research (Luxton et al., 2011; Pietrzak & McLaughlin, 2009). Outcome research on computerized interventions in general struggles with the resolution of methodological issues which are particularly salient to this emergent field (Postel et al., 2008; Kiluk et al., 2011). In addition, outcome research in suicide prevention is subject to strict ethical standards and faces the low base rate problem of suicide and suicidal behaviour (Gunnell & Frankel 1994; Lewis et al., 1997; Mishara & Weisstub, 2005).

Description of key services

Overview of 113Online services

113Online offers online preventive and therapeutic interventions to three target audiences: suicidal individuals, persons in their environment and those bereaved by suicide. Most services are offered 24/7 via the website www.113online.nl and by telephone. Help seekers can remain anonymous and pay no charges except for a 5 eurocents per minute telephone rate.

The 113Online services include:

- information, education and consultation,
- self-assessment tests,
- an online self-help course,
- moderated peer forums,
- chat and telephone hotlines, and
- online solution focused brief psychotherapy by chat and e-mail.

Organization and funding

In The Netherlands, in the period 1990 to 2005, the comparatively modest national suicide rate of 9.7 per 100,000 per year tended to be accepted as an unavoidable loss by policymakers and politicians. However, in 2005, prompted by advocacy organizations and opinion leaders, Parliament ordered a re-evaluation of the government policy (Bool et al., 2007). This created a window of opportunity for 113Online stakeholders to propose online suicide prevention as a policy priority (Loncke et al., 2011). With broad Parliamentary support, the Dutch Ministry of Health Care in 2008 provided a 2.2 million US dollar project grant for two years. After evaluation of the results, the project grant was transformed into a structural grant of 1 million US dollars per year.

Guiding principles and legal aspects

In designing the services, a number of guiding principles were defined. To engage the largest possible target audiences, services should be accessible with little or no requirements and with anonymity. The interventions should be evidence based, well tolerable and meeting the needs of the target audiences. All interventions and efforts should be aimed at facilitating talking about suicide, thus maximizing the opportunity to make contact with help seekers and help them survive. The Solution Focused Brief Therapy approach (SFBT; e.g. O'Connel, 2005; Bannink, 2007; Bakker & Bannink, 2008; MacDonald, 2011; Fiske, 2008) was chosen as a common therapeutic frame of reference to be used in all forms of direct work with help seekers, and in the language on the website.

Before starting the services, legal aspects had to be explored and addressed. Under Dutch law, online interventions are no different from regular interventions. The same rules and regulations apply. As in regular treatment, informed consent should be acquired. Offering online interventions to suicidal individuals is permitted when it is completely clear to help seekers what to expect and what not to expect from the service provider, and when all possible measures are taken to minimize unwanted effects and to optimize outcomes. Within this framework, 113Online found no significant legal obstacles. The liability insurance cost amounts to less than 10,000 US dollars per year.

Being a new health care organization, 113Online presented itself to the Dutch Health Care Inspectorate and obtained the legal status of licensed health care institution.

One important legal issue to address in this section is the extent to which 113Online is obliged to breach confidentiality and to initiate search and rescue operations. In the Netherlands, health care professionals are obliged to take protective measures and/or breach confidentiality when there is clear and present danger. In these instances 113Online can initiate search and rescue operations only when the help seeker complies with providing the practical information needed to locate him or her. Since most help seekers want to remain anonymous, this is often impossible. In order to get around this, 113Online has been providing police with IP addresses when a person's life is in danger. In one case, this has led to a timely location of the client and a rescue operation.

Practical aspects

113Online is based in a small office in Amsterdam, the Netherlands. Services are offered via www.113online.nl by the volunteers and professional staff of the 113Online Foundation. As of March 2013, the 113Online Foundation employed a professional staff of 12 full-time equivalent employees, including seven part-time therapists; a full-time general manager; a full-time web manager; a part-time research assistant, a part-time training coordinator and one part-time administrative collaborator. 113Online also employs three part-time volunteer therapists, and there are on average eight interns practicing online therapist skills under training and supervision of 113Online staff members.

During office hours, two or three therapists and three interns are on call in the 113Online office. Apart from performing therapy and consultation, they constitute the second line of help in crisis resolution, backing up the volunteers on the hotlines. They are in turn backed up by a psychiatrist who is available for therapist guidance by telephone. After office hours the professional duties are performed by members of the crisis resolution team of a large Amsterdam-based mental health organization.

113Online volunteers and employees collaborate not only in real time and face to face but also online, using a web-based digital working environment. This allows them to work on projects, to archive and update standards, to exchange information on clients and to share ideas. The digital workspace is especially suitable for quality control and education purposes. Volunteer intervision groups use this environment to upload chat logs and exchange peer feedback. Therapists use the environment to provide interns feedback and to uploaded chat therapy logs and therapy e-mails.

Key services

Information and education

Evidence-based education and practical information is presented on the website targeted at suicidal individuals, people concerned about someone and people bereaved by suicide. The 113Online educational information published on the site is supplemented by the possibility of consulting professionals with single questions via telephone or e-mail. Additionally, site visitors can use a directory of links to reliable sources of online information, education and self-help in a variety of problems areas.

The content of the educational material is aimed to help recognize suicidal ideation and despair, to foster hope, to enhance coping, to stimulate help seeking and to decrease isolation and taboos. The possibilities of coping and talking about suicidality and despair are stressed in order to attain the "Papageno-effect" (copycat behaviour of successful coping) (Niederkrotenthaler et al., 2010), and case examples of help seeking and survival are presented.

The 113Online educational material is worded in non-dramatic, sober and sensitive language. On the website, sentences are as short as possible to accommodate people with low education or reading problems. In line with the Solution Focused approach, positive terms are used (e.g.: "stay alive" instead of "not dying").

After a lengthy discussion, 113Online chose to use the Dutch word for suicide "zelfmoord" (self-murder) instead of the less current but more attenuating term "zelfdoding" (self-dying). Clearly the word "zelfmoord" has criminalizing connotations that may offend or hurt people, especially those who are bereaved. However, it is the common word for suicide in the Dutch language, whereas "Zelfdoding" is a politically correct term used mainly by professionals and officials. Additionally "Zelfdoding" is rarely used as a query in Internet browsers. The fact that several client focus groups advised to "walk the talk" of discussing suicide in a natural and straightforward manner was a decisive factor in the discussion. "If you don't dare to call 'zelfmoord' by its name, how can you expect us to feel free talking about it with you?" one focus group member put it succinctly.

Consultation

113Online offers professional advice via e-mail and telephone. This service is not aimed at acute crisis resolution or therapy, but at answering single questions. E-mails are answered within five working days. Telephone calls are taken during dedicated office hours. The consultation is offered by 113Online therapists, backed up by experienced psychiatrists. Topics include: how to find help, what to do when you are concerned someone you know may attempt suicide, what can be done about suicidal thinking and urges, and how to cope with bereavement after losing a loved one who died by suicide.

As with the education sections of the site, the consultation is based upon professional expertise, evidence and national guidelines. Help seekers are referred to offline and online resources including the 113Online services. In line with the disclaimers on the site, information about the limitations and drawbacks of online or telephone advice is communicated during the consultation process. Accordingly, no statements are made about formal psychiatric or somatic diagnoses; no advice is given regarding specific medications or ongoing treatments, and of course medication is not prescribed.

There are no restrictions as to who can ask for consultation and what this may be about, as long as the focus is suicide prevention and the consultation does not interfere with current treatments or working alliances with the help seekers' doctors or therapists. Questions that cross these lines are not discarded at once, but are explored in order to identify needs that can be met and answers that can be given within the realm of suicide prevention and the restrictions of the service.

Self-help course

To gain understanding of and control over suicidal ideation and rumination, help seekers can follow a six-module course based on cognitive behavioural therapy which is described in detail in another chapter in this book, "Reducing the burden of suicidal thoughts through online cognitive behavioural therapy self-help," by Kerkhof, van Spijker, and Mokkenstorm.

Self-tests

To obtain an instant impression of the severity of suicidal ideation, anxiety and depression, site visitors can fill out self-report questionnaires. Results are reported with automatically generated advice depending on the scores in relation to predetermined cut-off points marking levels of severity. Adults aged 23 years and older are offered the Beck Scale for Suicidal Ideation (BSS)(Beck & Steer, 1991), and the Depression and Anxiety Stress Scale (DASS-21) (Lovibond & Lovibond, 1995). Young individuals aged under 23 are offered modified versions of the Suicidal

Ideation Questionnaire-Junior (SIQ) (Reynolds, 1987); and the Hospital Anxiety and Depression Scale (Zigmond & Snaith, 1983).

Peer support

Service users are invited to share their experiences with 113Online on the homepage. These stories are publicly accessible, and are published to encourage site visitors to seek help. In addition, 113Online provides the opportunity to share thoughts, feelings and experiences on a moderated forum. Forum posts are monitored and moderated in order to prevent unwanted content from being published. The forum is accessible after registration and therefore not entirely public. A nickname and a working e-mail address are the minimal requirements for registration, allowing moderators to send direct messages to forum contributors to explain why posts have been removed.

Hotlines

113Online offers a 24/7 available telephone hotline and 13/7 available chat hotline, operated by volunteers recruited from the emotional support services Sensoor and Ex6. Sensoor is a large organization that provides attention and emotional support to those who need it. It is a member of Befrienders Worldwide and the International Federation of Telephone Emergency Services IFOTES. Ex6 is a smaller organization dedicated specifically to suicide prevention. Volunteers are largely based at their homes. Some Sensoor branches use central location from which volunteers operate the lines. The total volunteer capacity in March 2013 was 250, allowing for two to five volunteers per four-hour shift.

Volunteers working for 113Online are trained by psychologists in general counselling skills, suicidology, risk assessment and application of SFBT principles. Sensoor volunteers are supported and monitored by Sensoor trainers. Using an online working environment, Ex6 volunteers are organized in intervision groups with members offering online peer support and reviews of chat logs and telephone call reports. These intervision groups are supervised by professional coaches, performing quality checks to safeguard standards of work as defined in the service manual. During calls 113Online volunteers have instant access to assistance by 113Online professionals to whom callers can be transferred seamlessly.

Example: excerpt from a crisis chat

[13:26:30] anonymous: Ok, i tried to commit suicide in december and a few weeks ago

[13:26:38] anonymous: both failed

[13:26:54] anonymous: December with pills. Thought i had taken enough but no … .

[13:27:12] anonymous: few weeks ago after taking a load of pills i discovered … i have a longing.. to live after all.

[13:27:29] anonymous: now i do nothing else but think . how to take my life fast and painless

[13:29:28] Helper: Ok, a few weeks ago after a second attempt you discovered that you had a longing to live. Now you are thinking about taking your life fast and painlessly. Do I understand that your longing for life is still there but has gone to the background now?

[13:30:38] anonymous: yeah it is shifting … i have two sides i know … one side is desperate an powerless & wants get rid of the situation … and a side that wants to go for help

[13:30:45] anonymous: for therapy

[13:31:04] Helper: I see. I guess it is hard for you to experience this dilemma

[13:31:16] anonymous: the "healthy" side doesn't call anymore

[13:31:40] Helper: The side that wants help has become weaker?

[13:31:43] anonymous: yeah its a tough battle

[13:32:41] anonymous: i mean ivbeen in hospital for a while, later started somewhere else in therapy day treatment. That didn't help either.

[13:32:52] anonymous: they want me to do mbt, but before i can enter it'll be march next year.

[13:33:03] anonymous: in the meantime they want me to go into hospital again

[13:34:39] Helper: It is clear to me that you have been working hard to get a treatment that works well for you! I can imagine it is frustrating that you didn't get yet what you hoped for. Is that right?

[13:35:16] anonymous: That's right. bit by bit i lose hope. Hope to get better. Hope to get the right kind of help.

Psychotherapy

As a follow-up to crisis intervention or self-assessment, or after application via the website, 113Online offers suicidal clients solution focused brief therapy (SFBT). (Bannink, 2007). Clients can use chat or e-mail as a channel for therapeutic communication. Chat-therapy consists of a series of online sessions in which the patient-therapist dialogue is synchronous: they are connected online at the same time. This means that they have to make scheduled appointments. E-mail therapy is asynchronous: client and therapist exchange messages, typically not responding instantly but within days.

Results and experiences

In this section experiences and results will be reported on the usage, users and in the case of crisis chat the outcomes of key services.

Site visit: reach

Site visit data were generated using Google Analytics. Table 10.1 shows general site visit statistics of the period 5 September 2009 to 5 September 2012. In this period the site was visited 460,884 times by 236,153 unique visitors. Over half of the visitors is a returning visitor. The average number of page views per visit is 6.2. The average visit duration is almost 4 minutes per visit. Extrapolation of this 113Online visit statistics to the US ((Internet World Statistics, 2012): population of 313,232 million; with Internet penetration 78.3 per cent of households, leads to an expected 7000 visits per day in the USA.

Google Analytics page view statistics can be used to estimate the differential viewing of landing pages by the different target audiences. The period 1 sample (N = 117160 page views) was taken in the period from 7 October 2009 to 30 June 2011 with a cut-off dividing young and older visitors at age 22. The period 2 sample (N = 78404 page views) was taken in the period from 1 July 2011 to 7 September 2012 with a cut-off dividing young and older visitors at age 16 (see Table 10.2).

These findings defy a common assumption that 113Online encounters regularly, that its services are used predominantly by the young. But it is still impressive to see that one third of all views of the landing pages is apparently made by children 16 years of age or younger (see table 10.3).

Table 10.1   Site usage statistics

Site	Average per day
Site visits	420
Unique visitors	215
Page views	6.2
Visit duration	00:03:57

Site visitors: target audiences.

Site visitor patterns: "viewers", "clients", and "habitual users"

Site visit frequencies indicate visitor website usage patterns. According to their pattern three types of site visitors may be distinguished: "viewers", "clients", and "habitual users". "Viewers" are visitors that leave the site after taking a peak into "the shop". "Clients" are visitors who use the services of 113Online in a dedicated manner, but no longer than needed. "Habitual users" are visitors that are seemingly insatiable in using the site, without making progress, instigating a lower need of services offered. They visit the site every day, even more times a day, for prolonged periods.

Table 10.2 Pageview percentage per target audience

Page view Period 1 N = 117160	Young < 23	Older > 22	Young & Old
I am suicidal	20.1%	34.0%	54.10%
I am concerned	6.9%	12.2%	19.10%
I am bereaved	2.8%	8.5%	11.30%
In want information	4.8%	10.7%	15.50%
Total	34.60%	65.40%	100.00%
Page views Period 2 **N = 78408**	**Young** **< 17**	**Older** **> 16**	**Young** **& Old**
I am suicidal	14.5%	39.0%	53.50%
I am concerned	5.9%	15.5%	21.40%
I am bereaved	2.6%	7.4%	10.00%
In want information	6.6%	8.5%	15.10%
Total	29.6%	70.4%	100.0%

Table 10.3 Pageview percentage of young target audiences

Page	Pageviews Period 1	% < 23	Pageviews Period 2	% < 17
I am suicidal	63,300	20.1	41,927	14.5
I am concerned	22,440	6.9	16,791	5.9
I am bereaved	13,279	2.8	7842	2.6
I want information	18,141	4.8	11,848	6.6
Total	117,160	34.6	78,408	29.6

Table 10.4   Frequency of visits by unique visitors

Number of visits	Visitors	%
1	236,448	51.3
2	40,611	8.8
3	18,709	4.1
4–8	37,487	8.1
9–14	19,928	4.3
15–25	20,292	4.4
26–50	23,475	5.1
51–100	21,194	4.6
101–200	17,160	3.7
201+	25,580	5.6
Total	460,884	100.0

Table 10.4 shows the site visit frequency distribution of visitors in the period 5 September 2009 to 5 September 2012 as measured by Google Analytics. The largest proportion, almost 60 per cent of visits, is made by "viewers". After the initial one to three visits, a significant proportion of visitors starts using the site more regularly. Almost 22 per cent of site visits can be ascribed to regular use, with 4–50 site visits in three years. Among these visitors, most real "clients" can be expected; visitors that use the help offered effectively. At the current rate per day of 420 visits made by 215 unique visitors, this means that between 45 and 50 unique "clients" per day make effective use of 113Online services.

Almost 11 per cent of visits can be ascribed to intensive use, with over 50 visits in three years' time. Among these visitors there will be a population of "habitual users" with suicidal behaviours and interests defining an identity or a way of life. It is questionable to what extent 113Online services are helpful to them. The low access and anonymous services may even be harmful in sustaining behaviours that 113Online is trying to prevent. This warrants reflection on ways to seduce "habitual users" to become "clients". Possibly, a more assertive stance, for instance by active therapists' participation in forum discussions, may be a way to prevent the formation of an online suicidal identity among frequent users.

Types of users: "personae"

As 113Online service users are anonymous, it is hard to define user characteristics by measurement. However, based on their experiences with help seekers during their first three years, 113Online professionals have been able to establish typical profiles, or "personae", of help seekers in terms of acuity, help-seeking behaviour, needs and preferences.

In the target population of suicidal individuals, three prototypical personae were identified: Anne, Rick and Nina.

Anne is a 36-year-old depressed and acutely suicidal housewife, mother of two kids, husband often away from home. She is an introvert perfectionist, trying to fight her despair alone, not showing her feelings to others. Under a calm surface her feelings are a like a roller coaster. She has strong fantasies about taking her life to lessen the burden on others, sometimes including taking the lives of her children. She fears rejection and criticism, and is allergic to feeling more obligations. She needs validation, reassurance, advice, and support. She makes an excellent candidate for therapy.

Rick is a 20-year-old adolescent, recently abandoned by his girlfriend. She found him to be "too difficult". He is the youngest child of his parents, and still lives at home. He is an average type of guy, a little bland even, not sharing his deeper feelings with anyone. He is a thinker, wanting to analyze and understand everything. Sometimes he thinks himself to be a bit too autistic or intelligent for this world. He has exorbitantly high expectations of himself, but he is constantly ambivalent and unable to make decisions about school. He has failed his final undergraduate exams last year and has taken a "gap" year without knowing what to do with his time. He feels empty, a magnificent failure, an unnecessary organism on the face of the earth. He is ruminating about taking his life constantly in the past three weeks. Rick is a visitor of the 113Online site, contemplating whether he should send an application for therapy or the self-help course.

Nina is a 16-year-old sexually abused girl who self-harms frequently. She is, or has been, in various forms of treatment since her father left the family when she was 12. She has been diagnosed as having a borderline personality disorder and a post-traumatic stress disorder. She wets her bed regularly. At school she has been bullied because allegedly she smelled. In reaction, she has started to dress in "emo-gothic" style, wearing piercings and tattoos. She needs to talk, she wants to be taken very seriously and loses her temper easily, running away and making suicidal gestures. The most serious suicide attempt she made was by ingesting a television cable, hoping to perforate her intestines. She wants things to change, and sees no reason to make a change herself. She needs a lot of attention; it is rarely ever enough. Nina is a frequent user of the 113Online forum and of the crisis chat hotline.

These "personae" were used to target and market services on the website to individuals that can profit most from the care given. Having to optimize the use of a small capacity, choices have to be made which services to present in which manner to whom preferably. The "Nina" type of visitor is the most frequent and intensive user of the 113Online services. However, due to her treatment history, her externalizing attitude, and the fact that 113online is only one part of her "suicidal lifestyle," persons like Nina don't profit as much from the 113Online services as a "Anne" type of help seeker.

Also, reviewing "personae" in preparation of the website redesign described above, it became clear that one "persona" was missing: a middle aged, recently divorced, lonely, depressed and irritated male called "Joe". He has serious plans to commit suicide but also ambivalence because of his children and the hope things might work out with his ex-wife after all. He is disappointed by his general practitioner who did not ask about suicidality and proposed an antidepressant. Joe wants to shout and talk, but is afraid to cry. Writing about his sorrow and despair with someone on his side would be very helpful, making him a good candidate for e-mail therapy.

To make the site more appealing to "Joe" and "Anne" types of visitors (and less to the "Nina" type) their "personae" were translated into predicted site use preferences and behaviours. This resulted in a website redesign, with a new logo, new pictures, and a new user interface targeted to seduce more "Joe" and "Anne" type visitors to enter therapy while attracting "Rick" types to gradually use more self-help and perhaps later engage in more direct forms of communication with 113Online. At present there are no robust statistics to show the new website performance. A first impression is that the new, simplified design apparently seduces more visitors to become "clients," but that there is still work to motivate "habitual users" to become "clients" and use the opportunities to find new ways to cope instead of fostering old ones.

Self-test results

Adults

Suicidality

Adult site visitors were offered the 21-item BSS (Beck & Steer, 1991) as a suicidality self-test. In 2010 and 2011, 7381 visitors completed the BSS. This means on average per day the test is taken by 10 adults. This group consisted of 3011 males (41 per cent) and 4338 females (59 per cent), with a mean age of 37. Of the respondents 57 per cent had never attempted suicide, 22 per cent had attempted suicide once and 21 per cent had attempted suicide twice or more. Mean score was 19.8

(SD = 9.1); however, it was remarkable that a large proportion of persons either had the lowest score (0) or the highest (38), probably reflecting response set. When corrected for this phenomena, the mean score was 20.8 (SD = 7.7), resulting in a normal distribution of scores.

Based on the total score, the following automatically generated feedback was provided:

- 533 persons (7 per cent) scored 0–1 ("not suicidal").
- 129 persons (2 per cent) scored 2–3 ("mildly suicidal").
- 2900 persons (39 per cent) scored between 4–20 ("suicidal") and were advised to seek help.
- 3819 persons (52 per cent) scored between 21–38 ("severely suicidal") and were advised to seek help immediately.

Depression and anxiety

Adult site visitors were offered the 7-item DASS-21 as a self-test for anxiety and depression. 6050 persons completed the Depression and Anxiety Stress Scale (DASS-21) (Lovibond & Lovibond 1995) in 2010 and 2011: 2198 males (36 per cent) and 3791 females (63 per cent), with a mean age of 37. The mean score on the anxiety subscale was 19.7 (SD = 10.5) and 26.7 on the depression subscale (SD = 10.8). Scores on the anxiety subscale of 10 and up and 14 and up on the depression subscale indicated pathology.

Based on the scores on the anxiety and depression subscales, the following automatically generated feedback was provided:

- 640 persons (11 per cent) scored "relaxed".
- 159 persons (3 per cent) scored "anxious".
- 510 person (8 per cent) scored "depressed".
- 4741 persons (78 per cent) scored "anxious and depressed".

Youth

Suicidality

Young site visitors were offered a modified version of the 15-item SIQ-Junior. The original SIQ-Junior evaluates the severity and frequency of suicidal ideation amongst middle school students. On average six young visitors complete this test every day. In 2010 and 2011, 4521 young persons completed the suicidal ideation test, 1416 boys (31 per cent) and 3051 girls (68 per cent), with a mean age of 18 years. 43 per cent reported one or more suicide attempts. Based on the total score, the following automated feedback was given:

- 565 persons (13 per cent) probably were not suicidal.
- 229 persons (5 per cent) were mildly suicidal.
- 328 persons (7 per cent) were suicidal and were advised to seek help.
- 3399 persons (75 per cent) were severely suicidal and were advised to seek help immediately.

Anxiety and depression

Young site visitors were offered the 14-item Hospital Anxiety and Depression Scale (HADS) (Zigmond & Snaith, 1983) as a self-test for anxiety and depression. 4312 young persons completed the HADS, 1213 boys (28 per cent) and 3056 girls (71 per cent) with a mean age of 18. The mean score on the anxiety subscale was 12.4 (SD=2.7) and 11.0 (SD=5.4) on the depression subscale. Based on the total scores, the following automated feedback was given:

- 539 persons (12 per cent) were "relaxed".
- 646 persons (15 per cent) were "anxious".
- 208 persons (5 per cent) were "depressed".
- 2919 persons (68 per cent) were "anxious and depressed".

Hotline use

The usage of chat and telephone hotlines was retrieved from the website chat engine and telephone system database from 1 January 2012 to 31 August 2012. On average 113Online volunteers answer 34 acute chat calls in 13 hours per day and 16 telephone calls in 24 hours per day. The number of answered calls fluctuates with volunteer availability. It is clear that demand surpasses capacity, and that the demand for chat is greater than telephone.

Chat hotline: user characteristics and outcomes

To perform a preliminary study of the characteristics of chat hotline users and outcomes, a preliminary content analysis was performed from 1 June 2010 to 1 March 2011 using the logs of 4082 answered crisis chats with duration of longer than 7 minutes. A random sample (n=396) of chat call logs was drawn and analyzed. Each sampled chat log was reviewed by two members of a group of 18 trained and supervised master psychology students. Measures were: chat duration, apparent age and gender of caller, apparent presence of psychiatric problems and current psychiatric treatment status, and apparent (dis)satisfaction with the helper. The method developed by Mishara et al. (2007a; 2007b) in the silent monitoring study of US 1–800-SUICIDE network was used to assess the direction of change during a chat. The content of the first and last seven minutes of each chat call was scored according to a set of cognitive and emotional dimensions. One dimension was added: the degree to which the caller stated to be able to sustain his or her own thoughts.

The average chat duration was 61 min (SD 39). 48 per cent of chat callers could be identified as female, 15 per cent as male, and in 37 per cent of callers, gender could not be determined. The average age of callers mentioning their age (n=110) is 25.6. The oldest caller was 56, the youngest 12 years old. More than half of the callers was aged younger than 35 years. 46 per cent of callers reported to be in some form of mental health treatment. In 41 per cent of chat calls psychiatric symptoms and treatment were the main topics. Most callers were satisfied with the help: 63 per cent of callers thanked the helper spontaneously, 15 per cent of callers were dissatisfied.

Results of the outcome analysis are listed in Table 10.5. As a comparison, results earlier published by Mishara et al. (2007a; 2007b) were listed alongside the results of the current investigation.

Here we see that the outcomes of volunteer-operated 113Online chat hotlines and 1–800 telephone hotlines look alike. Both have a net positive effect, with states not changing during the call in about half of the calls. At the end of the call, 113Online callers seem to be a little bit happier and less depressed than 1–800 callers. On the other hand, they seem to be less resourceful than 1–800 callers, 15 per cent feeling more helpless at the end of the call. A remarkable finding is that in only 121 chat logs (31 per cent) a statement could be made about suicide

Table 10.5   Changes in feelings from the beginning to the end of chat sessions

1–800: n=1431 tel. calls 113: n=396 chats	Worse		No change		Better	
	1–800	113	1–800	113	1–800	113
Apprehensive/Confident	11%	7%	49%	52%	38%	43%
Sad/Happy	9%	5%	67%	51%	22%	44%
Helpless/Resourceful	10%	15%	41%	44%	49%	41%
Hopeless/Hopeful	11%	8%	47%	46%	40%	46%
Confused/Decided	10%	8%	36%	54%	52%	39%
Depressive mood	7%	8%	74%	56%	18%	36%
Desperate	6%	7%	77%	55%	16%	38%
Sustain thoughts		8%		56%		37%
Suicide ambivalence (n = 21)	2%	8%	84%	69%	14%	23%

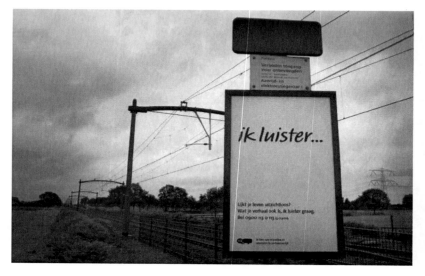

Figure 10.1   Railway Signpost: "I Listen"

ambivalence at the end of the call. This has resulted in adaptation of training and standards of volunteers, guiding them to ask about suicide ambivalence at the end of the call.

Railway related chat content

In 2011 the Dutch railway infrastructure company Prorail sought cooperation with 113Online. As a pilot, signposts reading "I Listen" referring to the availability of 113Online hotlines were erected along the railways on 9 "hotspot" locations. This was implemented during September 2011 (see figure 10.1).

To assess the presence of railway related content, and the impact of the "I Listen" signposts, chat logs were screened using the Microsoft Word search functionality. Search terms were: "rails", "railways", "train driver", "train", "station", "platform", "ProRail," "National Railways", and "conductor". Categories used were: the apparent distance of the caller in place and time to the railways at time of calling, apparent suicidal urges or plans involving the railways, and attitudes toward the use of the railways as a suicide method.

Chat logs were sampled in the period 1 October 2011 to 31 December 2011: 2853 chats by on estimate 1150 unique callers. In 260 chats

Table 10.6 Caller situations and attitudes in chats containing railway related content

Situation N = 260	N	% of 260
On the railway now	10	3.8
Today-yesterday	19	7.3
This week	10	3.8
Ever	27	10.3
Urge or a plan now	64	24.6
Decided against rail suicide	32	12.3
Ambivalent about rail suicide	23	8.8

(9.1 per cent) railway suicide related content was present. In 16 cases this related to someone else. Results are listed in Table 10.6.

In 10 cases, the caller was indicated to be on or very close the railways at the time of calling. This number is surprisingly high and has to be interpreted with caution. Technically, it is possible for users of modern smart phones to have a mobile chat, but it is also possible that these claims to be on the track might have been part of an urgent cry for help. 12.3 per cent (n = 45) indicated that they reject railway suicide, mentioning objections to this method such as the consequences for the train driver. Eighty-eight per cent (n = 23) indicated that they were ambivalent about railway suicide as a method.

A very positive finding is that in three months' time, and with sign posts at only hotspot locations, there were 3 direct and positive references to the " I Listen" signs, indicating that the caller had seen the signpost and aborted (preparations for) a suicide attempt. These findings have prompted erecting signposts to all hotspots in the Dutch railway network.

Experiences with online psychotherapy

The client demand for chat therapy is two to three times the demand for e-mail therapy, but the issues in chat and e-mail therapy are generally the same. The presenting problem of suicidality is often accompanied by a history of depression, anxiety, substance abuse, interpersonal conflict, loneliness and emptiness, shame and humiliation. An estimated 40 per cent receive mental health treatment elsewhere, and have sought help as a last resort or feeling needs that seem not to be met by their "regular" therapist. These patients often indicate having trouble talking about suicidality, in some cases because their therapist has allegedly defined suicide as a "non-issue". In these instances, 113Online aims at diminishing the presenting problem of suicidality, as well as developing ways the patient might reconnect with the therapist again about despair and self-harming thoughts.

113Online therapists view the outcomes of treatment as generally positive. Their overall impression is that the online therapy is at least stabilizing suicidal crises, allowing for ventilation of emotions and promoting resilience through the identification and implementation of adaptive coping strategies. The solution focused approach suits well to promote the sense of mastery and to reduce demoralization, while the patient is not growing dependent on therapists' views and advice. At termination of the contact, suicidality may still be present, but the patient knows how to cope with it (and with the underlying problems) better. Often they feel more free to seek help or support in their environment or in professional care. Due to the validation of pain and problems, as well as the compliments made for coping efforts and resilience, for many patients therapy is often a corrective emotional experience. As a result, the common problems of self-hate and low self-esteem are often decreased, levelling the field for self-protective behaviours and the adoption of safety plans.

Clients are offered up to eight e-mail therapy exchanges or chats sessions. A substantial number of patients disengage before any result can be achieved, sometimes to present themselves again, after prolonged periods of "radio silence" during which their therapist sends invitations to reconnect. The ambivalence of patients in help seeking does not only show in disengagement, but also in declining to be referred to offline forms of treatment at termination of the online therapy. In three years only 35 patients wanted to be referred to therapy following 113Online therapy. It seems that to many patients, referral to regular care evokes anxiety about losing autonomy and the potential to be disappointed. This finding has led to the adoption of a somewhat more supportive and directive stance, addressing these anxieties and motivating patients to seek help in regular care early in therapy.

In contrast with commonly heard professional opinions, but in line with research (Knaevelsrud & Maercker, 2006; Sucala et al., 2012) 113Online therapists find the lack of direct face-to-face contact not to interfere with the establishment of a meaningful therapeutic relationship. Perhaps on the contrary, the lack of direct face-to-face contact may be an advantage. Due to the online disinhibition effect (Suler, 2004), people may share more of their personal feelings online than they would in face-to-face contact. Working online, therapists manifest themselves through words only, restricting their display of competence and authority to the essence of their work: active listening and delivering the treatment. Knowing that the best thing they can do is perform therapy and use the therapeutic alliance to persuade people to take safety measures, it is easier to remain in a calm therapeutic stance even when the patient is very suicidal. This observation contradicts Lester's (2008) suggestion that therapists working with suicidal individuals online may become too anxious to be effective.

Forum

Forum use data are generated by Google Analytics and were sampled from 14 January 2010 to 14 September 2012. In this period a total of 99,375 messages on 2326 topics were posted – an average of 102.5 new posts and 2.4 new topics a day. The average duration of forum visits is 22 minutes, and the average number of posts read by forum visitors is 28. Because of the activity of spam bots and of visitors landing on the forum index page without entering the forum, the numbers of visits (191,613) and unique visitors (3659) in this period should be treated with caution. It is estimated that in any three-month period there are about 400 unique individuals visiting the forum regularly, of which 190 are "seeders", having posted more than one message. About 210 users are "leechers", reading but not posting messages. An estimated 120 unique visitors can be seen as intensive forum users, visiting the site every day.

Suicidal ideation was expressed in 15 per cent of posts, suicidal plans in 6 per cent. Initiators expressed suicidal thoughts and plans significantly more frequently than commenters. Also they displayed a negative or neutral mood significantly more frequently. Initiator content was dominated by negative feelings (81 per cent of their posts) and psychological complaints about (and problems with) mental health services (33 per cent).

Overall main content categories were: empathy and support (40 per cent) and self-disclosure (39 per cent). Advice was given in 170 posts, mainly by commenters. In 58 per cent of advice posts, the initiator did not respond; in 18 per cent the response indicated that the initiator found the advice to be not helpful; in 25 per cent the initiator indicated the advice to be helpful.

The general impression is that the forum allows for venting emotions and sharing problems to acquire peer support, advice and validation. It is unclear to what extent this influences suicidal behaviour or adaptive coping. However, 25 per cent of the peer advice given is well received and regarded as helpful. It is striking how many initiators complain about mental health services.

Moderating the forum has turned out to be quite demanding. It requires a continuous monitoring of new posts, which means a lot of reading. In addition, corresponding on moderator decisions with forum users is often complicated. Forum users regard the forum as "their" territory, their posts as their possessions, and monitoring as an infringement on their freedom of expression. More than once, discussions with single users on monitor decisions spilled over to the forum itself, kindling a negative mood among forum users.

These observations have led to the question to what extent 113Online professionals should participate in the forum, directly influencing discussions and responding to forum users. This would change the character of the forum from a peer support environment to a group therapy type of environment. This is a still ongoing discussion.

Adverse events: suicides

In the past three years, three suicides of 113Online help seekers occurred. It is possible that more suicides have occurred that were not reported to us. In all cases the help seeker turned out to be female and in treatment in regular mental health care as well. One suicide was a forum user, for whom an obituary was posted on the forum. One suicide was a woman just starting 113Online e-mail therapy, and one a woman who had received six e-mail therapy exchanges. In both cases their family had searched the computer of the deceased and found references to visits to the113Online website in the Internet search history. They contacted 113Online to inform the organization about the suicide and shared their appreciation for our work.

Psychological autopsy analysis of the suicides revealed that the deceased help seekers had been contemplating suicide for a long time. There were no reasons to assume that the quality of care provided by 113Online had been insufficient. 113Online reported the suicides to the national Dutch Health Care Inspectorate, which accepted these without further inquiry or comments.

Discussion and future directions

Reach and access

The analysis of page views to the landing pages indicate that 113Online reaches the target audiences (suicidal individuals, concerned, bereaved). According to the self-test outcomes, site visitors suffer moderate to (sometimes extremely) severe suicidal ideation, anxiety and depression.

This means that 113Online reaches a significant population with clinical levels of psychopathology.

Acceptability

An estimated 60 per cent of 113Online help seekers appear not to be in regular care while suffering severe mental health problems and suicidality. These help seekers view 113Online as an acceptable alternative to regular, face-to-face health care. Their concern that seeking help may complicate things and add to the pain is often encountered. Patients often fear restrictive measures, criticism, naïve optimism and coercion to keep on living being imposed on them as a consequence of seeking help. As 113Online workers have learned from patients: to them the perspective of suicide may seem safer than the perspective of being helped. Their definition of safety is being free from the (fear of) pain. This is not necessarily what helpers want them to do: stay alive.

These observations explain why 113Online reaches people who have not been reached by regular care services. Online, there is more autonomy, more control and less shame. Therefore, many patients feel safer and more at ease seeking help online than face to face. Together with the practicality of the Internet, its ubiquitous presence and geographical independence, this lowers the barriers to seek help. In addition, the solution focused approach of 113Online amplifies engagement of reluctant help seekers that want to stay in control but need validation and a way to find alternative solutions they can apply. In this manner 113Online provides a supplementary health care environment for people who would otherwise shy away from help.

As observed in the content analysis of forum and crisis chats, help seekers that do receive regular treatment often express dissatisfaction with their treatment or their therapist. This may be interpreted as a sign of ineffectiveness of treatment in regular care, leaving the patient in despair about agonizing (often chronic) symptoms not responding to treatment. It may also be a sign of dissatisfaction with therapists' handling of suicidal thoughts and behaviours, e.g. their ability to validate and explore suicidality in a professional and therapeutic way. This may be true as many clinicians recognize a lack of training and a degree of tension working with suicidal patients (Aish et al., 2000; Wasserman & Wasserman, 2009; Scheerder, 2009). Another plausible interpretation is that the dissatisfaction constitutes a reaction to limit setting or neglecting self-harm habits as is practiced in the treatment of borderline patients. Another possible explanation is that some suicidal patients have a tendency to be negative with any experience, perhaps as a result of their depression, and therefore are negative about health care as well. Probably in each case an individual mix of these possible explanations may play a role.

The overall impression is that the involvement of 113Online with a patient in ongoing offline treatment does not cause undesired developments or outcomes to occur. In many cases it has led to greater satisfaction with regular treatment.

Effectiveness

The main question still remains unanswered: Is 113Online effective in preventing suicide? The experiences and preliminary results presented are promising. Crisis chats appear to have a positive effect on one third of callers, while half of them are unaffected but not worsened. Anecdotal therapist reports indicate that help seekers profit from brief online therapy and professional online crisis interventions. There are very impressive findings that erecting signposts along railways has resulted in abortion of intended suicide attempts and the initiation of help seeking. However, these promising findings have to be confirmed by more research. Different research approaches can be taken. Conducting a descriptive and naturalistic study using systematically recorded outcome measures or other ratings of change will give a more objective description of the experiences and observations presented in this chapter. The best way to identify the effect of treatment is performing a randomized controlled trial. At present, preparations are being made to perform an experimental study of the effect of 113Online solution focused brief therapy compared to treatment as usual.

Conclusion

113Online demonstrates the feasibility, acceptability and accessibility of a wide range of online preventive and therapeutic interventions offered to a population of (often severely) suicidal and individuals. 113Online provides an alternative gateway to care for suicidal individuals that shy away from help in regular offline care. It provides a temporary supplement for patients with needs unmet in ongoing regular treatment, helping them to deal with this with their offline therapist. Online intervention permits the performance of content analyses on the communication of suicidal individuals, providing a unique insight into relevant aspects of suicidal behaviour and help seeking. The positive impression of the effectiveness of 113Online in preventing suicide and in promoting resilience and coping needs to be confirmed by future research.

References

Aish, A. M., Ramberg, I. L., & Wasserman, D. (2002). Measuring attitudes of mental health-care staff towards suicidal patients. *Archives of Suicide Research, 6*(4), 309–323.

Andrews, G., Cuijpers, P., Craske, M. G., McEnvoy, P., & Totov, N. (2010). Computer therapy for the anxiety and depressive disorders is effective, acceptable and practical health care: A meta-analysis. *PLOS ONE, 5*(10), 1–6.

Baker, D., & Fortune, S. (2008). Understanding self-harm and suicide websites: A qualitative interview study of young adult website users. *Crisis, 29*(3), 118–122.

Bakker, J. M., & Bannink, F. P. (2008). Oplossingsgerichte therapie in de psychiatrische praktijk. *Tijdschrift voor Psychiatrie, 50*(1), 55–59.

Bannink, F. P. (2007). Solution-focused brief therapy. *Journal of Contemporary Psychotherapy, 37*, 87–94.

Barak, A. (2007). Emotional support and suicide prevention through the internet: A field project report. *Computers in Human Behavior, 23*(2), 971–84.

Beck, A. T., & Steer, R. A. (1991). *Beck scale for suicide ideation manual.* San Antonio: The Psychological Corporation.

Biddle, L., Gunnell, D., Owen-Smith, A., Potokar, J., Longson, D., Hawton, K., Kapur, N., & Donovan, J. (2012). Information sources used by the suicidal to inform choice of method. *Journal of Affective Disorders, 136*, 702–709.

Bool, M., Blekman, J., de Jong, S., Ruiter, M., & Voordouw, I. (2007). *Verminderen van Suïcidaliteit: Actualisering van het Advies Inzake Suïcide, Gezondheidsraad 1986 (Reducing suicide: Policy advice actualization of the 1986 Health Council advice regarding suicide).* Utrecht, The Netherlands: Trimbos Institute.

Bruffaerts, R., Demyttenaere, K., Hwang, I., Chio, W. T., Sampson, N., Kessler, R. C., ... Nock, M. K. (2011). Treatment of suicidal people around the world. *The British Journal of Psychiatry, 199*, 64–70.

Cuijpers, P., Boluijt, P., & van Straten, A. (2008). Screening of depression in adolescents through the Internet: Sensitivity and specificity of two screening questionnaires. *European Child & Adolescent Psychiatry, 17*(1), 32–38.

Durkee, T., Hadlaczky G., Westerlund, M., & Carli, V. (2011). Internet pathways in suicidality: A review of the evidence. *International Journal of Environmental Research Public Health, 8*(10), 3938–3952.

Fiske, H. (2008). *Hope in action. Solution-focused conversations about suicide.* New York: Routledge.

Gould, M. S., Munfakh J. L., Kleinman, M., & Lake, A. M. (2012). National suicide prevention lifeline: Enhancing mental health care for suicidal individuals and other people in crisis. *Suicide and Life-Threatening Behavior, 42*(1), 22–35.

Gunnell, D., Bennewith, O., Kapur, N., Simkin, S., Cooper, C., & Hawton, K. (2012). The use of the Internet by people who die by suicide in England: A cross sectional study. *Journal of Affective Disorders, 141*(1–2), 480–483.

Gunnell, D., & Frankel, S. (1994). Prevention of suicide: Aspirations and evidence. *BMJ, 308*, 1227–1233.

Harris, K. M., McLean, J. P., & Sheffield, J. (2009). Examining suicide-risk individuals who go online for suicide-related purposes. *Archives of Suicide Research, 13*(3), 264–276.

Hengeveld, M. W., Kerkhof, A. J. F. M., & van der Wal, J. (1988). Evaluation of psychiatric consultations with suicide attempters. *Acta Psychiatrica Scandinavica*, *77*(3), 283–289.

Internet World Statistics. (2012). Retrieved 26 September 2012 http://www.internetworldstats.com.

Kiluk, B. D., Sugarman, D. E., Nich, C., Gibbons, C. J., Martino, S., Rounsaville, B. J., & Caroll, K. M. (2011). A methodological analysis of randomized clinical trials of computer-assisted therapies for psychiatric disorders: Towards improved standards for an emerging field. *The American Journal of Psychiatry*, *168*(8), 790–799.

Knaevelsrud, C., & Maercker, A. (2006). Does the quality of the working alliance predict treatment outcome in online psychotherapy for traumatized patients? *Journal of Medical Internet Research*, *8*(4), e31.

Krysinska, K. E., & De Leo, D. (2007). Telecommunication and suicide prevention: hopes and challenges for the new century. *Journal of Death & Dying*, *55*(3), 237–253.

Lester, D. (2008). The use of the Internet for counseling the suicidal individual: Possibilities and drawbacks. *Omega*, *58*(3), 233–250.

Lewis, G., Hawton, K., & Jones, P. (1997). Strategies for preventing suicide. *British Journal of Psychiatry*, *171*, 351–354.

Loncke, M., Ngo, T., & Nauta, F. (2011). Prima Praktijken: 113Online. Anonymous online help to prevent suïcide. (Anonieme online hulpverlening bij suïcidepreventie). *Lectoraat Innovatie in de Publieke sector*. http://www.lectoraatinnovatie.nl/wp-content/uploads/2009/03/113-Online-eindversie.pdf

Lovibond, S. H., & Lovibond, P. F. (1995). *Manual for the Depression Anxiety Stress Scales* (2nd ed.). Sydney: Psychology Foundation of Australia.

Luxton, D. D., June, J. D., & Kinn, J. T. (2011). Technology-based suicide prevention: Current applications and future directions. *Telemedicine and e-Health*, *17*(1), 50–54.

MacDonald, A. (2011). Solution-Focused Therapy: Theory, Research & Practice (2nd rev. ed.). London: Sage Publication Ltd.

McGinty, K. L., Saeed, S., Simmons, S. C., & Yildirim, Y. (2006). Telepsychiatry and e-mental health services: Potential for improving access to mental health care. *Psychiatric Quarterly*, *77*(4), 335–342.

Mishara, B. L., Chagnon, F., Daigle, M., Balan, B., Raymond, S., Marcoux, I., … Berman, A. (2007a). Which helper behaviors and intervention styles are related to better short-term outcomes in telephone crisis intervention? Results from a silent monitoring study of calls to the U.S. 1–800- SUICIDE network. *Suicide Life-Threatening Behavior*, *37*(3), 291–307.

Mishara, B. L., Chagnon, F., Daigle, M., Balan, B., Raymond, S., Marcoux, I., … Berman, A. (2007b). Comparing models of helper behavior to actual practice in telephone crisis intervention: A silent monitoring study of call to the U.S. 1–800-SUICIDE network. *Suicide Life-Threatening Behavior*, *37*(3), 308–321.

Mishara, B. L., & Weisstub, D. N. (2005). Ethical and legal issues in suicide research. *International Journal of Law and Psychiatry*, *28*(1), 23–41.

Niederkrotenthaler, T., Voracek, M., Herberth, A., Till, B., Strauss, M., Etzersdorfer, E., Eisenwort, B., & Sonneck, G. (2010). Role of media reports in completed and prevented suicide: Werther v. Papageno effects. *The British Journal of Psychiatry*, *197*(3), 234–243.

O'Connel, B. (2005). *Solution-focused therapy*. London: Sage Publications Ltd.

Pagura, J., Fotti, S., Katz, L. Y., & Sareen, J. (2009). Help seeking and perceived need for mental health care among individuals in Canada with suicidal behaviors. *Psychiatric Services, 60*(7), 943–949.

Pietrzak, E., & McLaughlin, R. (2009). *The effectiveness of online suicide prevention programs: A literature review*. Queensland, Australia: Centre for Military and Veterans' Health.

Pirkis, J., Burgess, P., Meadows, G., & Dunt, D. (2001). Self-reported needs for care among persons who have suicidal ideation or who have attempted suicide. *Psychiatric Services, 52*(3), 381–383.

Pitman, A., & Osborn, D. P. J. (2011). Cross-cultural attitudes to help-seeking among individuals who are suicidal: New perspective for policy-makers. *British Journal of Psychiatry, 199*(1), 8–10.

Postel, M. G., de Haan, H. A., & de Jong, C. A. J. (2008). E-therapy for mental health problems: A systematic review. *Telemedicine and e-Health, 14*(7), 707–715.

Reynolds, W. M. (1987). *Suicidal Ideation Questionnaire-Junior*. Odessa, FL: Psychological Assessment Resources.

Saini, P., Windfuhr, K., Pearson, A., Da Cruz, D., Miles, C., While, D., ... Kapur, N. (2010). Suicide prevention in general care: General practitioners' views on service availability. *BMC Research Notes, 3*, 246.

Sarchiapone, M., Temnik, S., & Carli, V. (2009). Preventing suicide through the Internet. In Sher, L., & Vilens, A. (eds), *Internet and suicide* (pp. 99–115). New York: Nova Science Publishers Inc.

Scheerder, G. (2009). *The care of depression and suicide: Attitudes, skills, and current practices of community and health professionals* (Doctoral dissertation). Katholieke Universiteit Leuven, Leuven, Belgium.

Spek, V., Cuijpers, P., Nyklicek, I., Riper, H., Keyzer, J., & Pop, V. (2007). Internet-based cognitive behaviour therapy for symptoms of depression and anxiety: A meta-analysis. *Psychological Medicine, 37*(3), 319–328.

Sucala, M., Schnur, J. B., Constantino, M. J., Miller, S. J., Brackman, E. H., & Montgomery, G. H. (2012). The therapeutic relationship in e-therapy for mental health: A systematic review. *Journal of Medical Internet Research, 14*(4), e110.

Suler, J. (2004). The online disinhibition effect. *Cyberpsychological Behaviour, 7*(3), 321–326.

Taylor, T. L., Hawton, K., Fortune, S., & Kapur, N. (2009). Attitudes towards clinical services among people who self-harm: Systematic review. *British Journal of Psychiatry, 194*(2), 104–110.

Ten Have, M., Dorsselaer, S., Tuithof, M., & de Graaf, R. (2011). Nieuwe gegevens over suïcidaliteit in de bevolking (New data on suicidality in the population). Resultaten van de "Netherlands Mental Health Survey and Incidence Study (NEMESIS-2). Trimbos Instituut.

Wasserman, D., & Wasserman, C. (2009). *Oxford textbook of suicidology and suicide prevention: A global perspective*. Oxford: Oxford University Press.

Zigmond, A. S., & Snaith, R. P. (1983). The Hospital Anxiety and Depression Scale. *Acta Psychiatrica Scandinavica, 67*(6), 361–370.

11

Suicide Bereavement Online: Sharing Memories, Seeking Support, and Exchanging Hope

Karolina Krysinska and Karl Andriessen

Over the last three decades, due to its increasing availability and ease of use, Internet has become the important source of (mental) health information and support. For instance, in 2010, 80 per cent of US Internet users looked for online information regarding specific diseases or treatments, 18 per cent searched online for someone who shared similar health concerns, and 15 per cent found health information on social network sites (Pew Research Center, 2011). Also the bereaved, including those bereaved by suicide, who are often identified as "suicide survivors", turn to online resources such as forums, chats and online memorials to better cope with their loss. Indeed, the Internet has an enormous potential to become a valuable resource for the bereaved by providing bereavement-related support (such as opportunities for sharing information and networking), bereavement-related activities, such as memorialization (e.g., online cemeteries), and professional psychological interventions (Stroebe, van der Houwen, & Schut, 2008). This chapter provides an overview of online resources available to the bereaved after suicide, advantages and challenges of seeking support and information on the Internet, as well as major features of computer-mediated communication. The online resources most frequently used by the bereaved (and most frequently studied by researchers), such as peer support groups, online memorials and social networking sites are presented in more detail, along with evidence regarding their impact on the grief process. Finally, the issue of quality and trustworthiness of online information for the bereaved is discussed and recommendations for development of a user-friendly and professional website are provided.

Seeking online support in bereavement

Why go online for information and support in bereavement?

A wide range of online mental health resources, including resources for the bereaved, is available for those seeking information and support. Although a detailed discussion of the prerequisites, advantages and disadvantages of different types of online resources and services is beyond the scope of this chapter, in general, online material can be divided into three broad categories: passive, active and interactive (Schalken et al., 2010). Passive online resources include websites containing information, tips and advice, links, Frequently Asked Questions, testimonials and news/media reports. For example, information for the bereaved by suicide is provided online by Befrienders Worldwide (www.befrienders.org), the American Association of Suicidology (www.suicidology.org/suicide-survivor-resources) and Healthtalkonline in the UK (www.healthtalkonline.org). The use of passive resources requires minimum effort; nonetheless the bereaved have to be able to find the website, evaluate its usefulness and effectively use the available information (i.e., digital literacy). Active resources, such as online self-tests, multiple choice tests, and other insight instruments allow the users to better understand the seriousness of their problem and/or the type of help most suited to their needs. For example, Rouw.nl, an online funeral service in the Netherlands, allows the bereaved to take a self-test measuring complicated grief (www.rouw.nl/rouwmeter/). Some active websites allow uploading personal testimonials which can be shared with other users of the site. This type of resources require the user's involvement and readiness to share personal information, such as answering a series of personal questions regarding the nature of loss, and emotional, cognitive and behavioural reactions, which may lead to resistance and anonymity/confidentiality concerns (Schalken et al., 2010).

Interactive resources include professional protocol-based psychological treatments for complicated grief (e.g., Wagner, Knaevelsrud, & Maercker, 2006), psychoeducational programs for the bereaved (e.g., Dominick et al., 2009–2010), asynchronous online forums, email help and step-by-step programs, and synchronous one-on-one or group chats. Examples of online forums for the bereaved by suicide are the Internet Communities of Parents of Suicides and Friends & Families of Suicides (http://health.groups.yahoo.com) and the Circle Discussion Board of Survivors of Suicide (www.survivorsofsuicide.com/wwwboard.html) in the US, as well as a forum for suicide survivors in Flanders (Belgium) available at the website of Werkgroep Verder (www.werkgroepverder.be).

The use of interactive resources might require serious investment of time and energy, sharing personal details and, in case of online therapy and other professional treatments, giving up anonymity (Schalken et al., 2010). In addition, other types of online sites, such as social networks, online memorials and blogs can be used by the bereaved in order to better cope with their loss (Sofka, Noppe Cupit, & Gilbert, 2012).

There are many reasons why individuals, including the bereaved after suicide, choose to use online resources. Online bereavement-related activities allow both seeking and maintaining contact with other bereaved, and continuing bonds and communication with the deceased (Roberts, 2004; Sofka et al., 2012). Finding others in the digital space who have gone through a similar experience of loss provides a unique chance to share one's story in a safe and empathic environment. Given the taboo nature of loss by suicide and the social stigma surrounding suicide, online information and help might be particularly attractive to survivors who are often bereft of other support (Berger, Wagner, & Baker, 2005; Grad, 2011).

Online help might be of special appeal to the "digital natives" – adolescents and young adults, as well as people with physical handicaps, such as mobility or hearing problems. Online contact, due to the reduced communication channels, might be the medium of choice for those who prefer to write rather than to talk, and those who are afraid or ashamed to show emotions or to cry during a face-to-face contact. Online information, support and services are available over geographical and national borders, and might be the only resource for those who live in rural and remote areas or other regions where face-to-face help is non-existent (Bocklandt, 2011; Van Hecke, 2012).

Generally, online resources are available 24/7, anonymously and without the mediation of the third parties, such as referral from a general practitioner or guidance from a mental health professional. These factors can significantly reduce the resistance to seek help among individuals who due to privacy and anonymity concerns avoid regular mental health services. Participants of online peer support groups, chats, online crisis intervention or therapy often have more control over the process and content of the helping intervention than those who use face-to-face facilities. They can easier decide when to initiate and to break contact, and which content should be shared with others. Nonetheless, due to potentially lower involvement and the ease of ending contact without warning, the drop-out rate in an online treatment or peer contact is often higher than in a face-to-face interaction. Suddenly breaking contact is especially poignant in case of synchronous one-on-one communication, such as a chat (Bocklandt, 2011).

Can the bereaved find helpful information and support online?

What kind of online resources are available to suicide survivors?

Anecdotal and clinical observations, supported by accumulating research evidence, show that the bereaved use the Internet to share their grief and to connect with others, and to maintain their relationship with the deceased . Already almost a decade ago Vanderwerker and Prigerson (2004) found that approximately half of the bereaved in the USA used Internet and/or email, and that such online resources seemed to improve their quality of life and could protect against mental problems secondary to bereavement. More recent data show that more than half of the bereaved in North America are currently using online mutual bereavement support, such as email lists, Internet forums and/or chat rooms (often in combination), while one in five bereaved used such support in the past (van der Houwen et al., 2010b). A study conducted in the UK addressed specifically the use of the Internet by the bereaved by suicide (Chapple & Ziebland, 2011). It showed that suicide survivors use the Internet to find practical information, to inform friends and family about the death, to get online peer support from other bereaved, and to memorialize the deceased through an online memorial. Despite the abundance and popularity of bereavement-related online material, not much is known about resources available specifically for suicide survivors. In order to fill in this gap an Internet search study using several popular search engines was conducted to see what type of resources people bereaved by suicide are likely to find online and to describe the quality of such resources (Krysinska & Andriessen, 2010).

Altogether the searches retrieved 145 websites, and this diverse material encompassed personal websites created by suicide survivors themselves, sites developed by bereavement support groups, crisis intervention and mental health services, suicide prevention organizations and help lines, as well as academic and research institutions and educational organizations. Only a relatively modest number of the retrieved websites was created by professional bereavement and suicide prevention organizations and services. For example, the International Association for Suicide Prevention website came up only 14 times in 520 searches, including 10 hits when the search term was "(suicide) postvention". National suicide bereavement organizations such as Compassionate Friends in Canada, Console in Ireland, and Cruse Bereavement Care in the UK came up only seven, three and one time, respectively. A similar observation was made by Recupero, Harms and Noble (2008) in a study on suicide information available online: mental health organizations' websites were not frequently found through the searches, and the authors suggested implementation of search engine optimization strategies to increase the likelihood of retrieval of professional and trustworthy websites. It is also important to add that the searches did not retrieve websites and resources which seemed to be offensive or potentially harmful to the bereaved.

The content and quality analysis of the fifteen most frequently retrieved websites ("top fifteen") showed differences in regards to the recency and amount of information presented, the way the websites were organized and the search terms needed to find the site. Despite such differences, the majority of the sites contained information on suicide bereavement and suicide, referral information for people at risk of suicide and for people bereaved by suicide, resources (such as suggested reading, leaflets and material for sale) and links to other relevant websites. Almost half of the websites also provided opportunities for interactive communication. Nonetheless, the analysis of the "top fifteen" websites found only one site linked to professional e-help and none of them had a HONcode certificate (Health on the Net Foundation, 2012), i.e. trustworthiness certificate awarded to medical and health websites which meet seven quality criteria discussed in more detail later in this chapter.

It is interesting that the majority of referral resources for the bereaved by suicide which were listed and recommended on the personal bereavement websites analysed among the "top fifteen" sites were face-to-face suicide bereavement support groups, and often a US website had a link to the online support group directory of the American Foundation for Suicide Prevention (www.afsp.org). Very few websites provided information or encouragement for seeking help from mental health professionals and services or general practitioners.

Online support groups

Seeking help and support in a group of individuals who share a similar experience of a medical illness, mental health problems, an addiction, trauma or loss has become a popular manner of coping with the challenges of life and negative life events (Davison, Pennebaker, & Dickerson, 2000; King & Moreggi, 2007). Over the last two decades the Internet has become a meeting place for people seeking peer support via mailing lists, newsgroups, discussion forums and live chat rooms

(Eysenbach et al., 2004; Tanis, 2007). The bereaved, including suicide survivors, are no exception; face-to-face or online peer support has been a treatment of choice for many people not willing or not being able to engage in a helping relationship with a professional (Feigelman et al., 2008; Hollander, 2001). The potentially non-stop access to online support, anonymity, not feeling comfortable sharing grief with family and friends, and finding empathy, validation and understanding in an online group are the most important reasons why suicide survivors and other bereaved choose to participated in online groups (Chapple & Ziebland, 2011; Feigelman et al., 2008; Oliveri, 2003). It has been observed that online grief support groups are more popular among women, especially young women, than men and their participants often also seek face-to-face professional or peer support (Chapple & Ziebland, 2011; Feigelman et al., 2008).

A qualitative study by Swartwood, McCarthy Veach, Kuhne, Lee and Ji (2011) of the online forum messages exchanged by the bereaved provides an interesting insight into the content and dynamics of the online communication and peer support (unfortunately the study did not extract content specific to communication between suicide survivors and/or the bereaved by suicide with other bereaved). Four major themes, which together can be summarized as "exchange of hope", were found: sharing one's personal story, validating the grief experience, offering psychosocial support, and sharing information and resources. Sharing one's story often took place in response to a posted message and followed a certain informal standard. It usually started with an acknowledgement of the other person's loss (e.g., "I am sorry to hear about your loss."), followed by a description of one's own loss experience and emotional reactions (e.g., "My child died as well. Here is my story ..."), and ended with advice or comforting words (e.g., "Please continue to write about your story. It helps. I will be thinking about you."). Validation of the grief experience included normalization of the reactions of the other bereaved and permission to feel and to behave in the way which felt natural to the person without guilt, shame of social stigma (e.g., "What you describe is normal. Give it time just take the time you need for yourself right now."). The forum members offered each other psychosocial support by attending to the emotional difficulties of the others and creating an atmosphere of acceptance and understanding. Last but not least, the bereaved exchanged information about the process of grieving itself (e.g., expected duration, psychological reactions), available resources, such as peer support groups, organizations, websites, books, music or poetry. They also shared advice how to cope with the loss, including encouragement of self-care activities (e.g., "Come to this site when you want to cry.") and religious consolation (e.g., "You will be in my prayers.").

Online memorials

Online memorials are webpages or websites dedicated to honouring the dead and are usually used as a supplement to traditional bereavement rituals (De Vries & Moldaw, 2012; Roberts, 2004). They are usually created by family members (parents, children) or friends by the deceased, although there are also websites created by funeral homes and other commercial organizations. Online memorials include freestanding webpages dedicated to the deceased (e.g., a list of memorials at http://childsuicide.homestead.com/MemorialSites.html), webrings in which individual webpages sharing a common theme such as cause of death or relationship with the deceased are linked together (e.g., a webring of suicide memorial sites at http://hub.webring.org/hub/suicidehurts), web cemeteries (e.g., the suicide memorial at the World Wide Cemetery at /www.cemetery.org/Memorials/suicide.html) and formalized online memorial sites (e.g., the Suicide Memorial Wall at www.suicidememorialwall.com).

Online memorials are usually created and maintained along with a physical grave, although sometimes due to geographical distance or the nature of loss, especially in case of socially unacceptable or unrecognized relationship with the deceased (i.e., disenfranchised grief), they may be a replacement for a traditional grave. Type, content and format of online memorials differ (De Vries & Rutherford, 2004; Roberts & Vidal, 2000). They range from personal letters to the deceased to formal eulogies, obituaries or tributes, and usually contain expressions of sadness, themes of reunion, religious references, philosophical musings about life and death, and the belief that the deceased is watching over the activities of the living. While some online memorial sites or web cemeteries have an uniform format, for example, only the name and birth and death dates are presented (e.g., the Suicide Memorial Wall at http://www.suicidememorialwall.com), others allow a more individualized approach and the bereaved can upload photos, videos, flowers, poems, music or digital candles (e.g., the suicide memorial at the World Wide Cemetery at http://www.cemetery.org/Memorials/suicide.html).

On the one hand, online memorials allow continuing bonds with the deceased (De Vries & Rutherford, 2004; Roberts, 2004; Roberts & Vidal, 2000). They can be established many years after the death, for example, one study showed that 7 per cent of online memorials were created more than 20 years after the loss (Roberts & Vidal, 2000). Online memorials are often regularly visited and tended with love and care just like traditional burial sites. In a study by Roberts (2004), 74 per cent of the bereaved who created an online memorial visited it daily in the 1st month, 68 per cent visited it at least weekly in the 1st year, and 91 per cent revised the memorial adding new or additional elements. For some bereaved, online memorialization may be a way to communicate with the deceased via online messages or letters describing recent life events or changes, such as birth of a child or moving home. On the other hand, online memorialization allows sharing the grief experience with the living (De Vries & Rutherford, 2004; Roberts, 2004; Roberts & Vidal, 2000). The bereaved can share their memories of the deceased, receive or show signs of compassion through signing online guestbooks, leaving digital flowers or burning digital candles. Online memorials can be created, maintained or visited with others, and letting others know about the memorial can be an opportunity to talk about the death with those who knew the deceased as well as strangers.

Roberts and Vidal (2000) in their study of four online cemeteries identified 10 per cent of online graves as devoted to people who took their own lives (this percentage is only an estimation: the cause of death was mentioned only in one third of the analyzed memorials). Online memorials created by those bereaved by suicide, as well as memorials devoted to victims of other sudden and/or violent deaths, seem to have unique features (De Vries & Rutherford, 2004; Roberts & Vidal, 2000). They include information about the cause of death more often than other memorials, contain more often a wish that the deceased might (finally) rest in peace, as well as attempts to understand and to come to terms with the death (e.g., "Ten years ago you decided to leave us of your own will. Today I finally respect your decision even if I will still grieve for you and I don't understand it."; GR, 1997 in Roberts & Vidal, 2000; p. 52).

Social networks

The popularity of social networks has been increasing rapidly, and as of April 2012, there were 901 million active Facebook users worldwide (Socialbakers, 2012). In the US, 66 per cent of the online population, or in other words, 157 million people, have joined this networking site and, according to estimations, 375,000 US Facebook users die every year (Health Service Executive, 2011). Given the need to deal with the digital legacy left behind by the deceased, Facebook has introduced a set of procedures for creating a "memorial profile" (more information about memorializing an account is available at the Facebook Help Center at www.facebook.com/help).

Given the popularity of social networking sites among adolescents and young adults, some studies have looked at how such sites are used after the death of a peer and the impact of this type of digital legacy on the young bereaved, including suicide survivors (Hiefje, 2012; Williams & Merten, 2009). The sites turned out to be important means of continuing the relationship and communicating with the deceased; many bereaved peers posted messages addressed to the deceased friend. The sites helped to commemorate the lost friend and to keep connected with him or her, as well as the other bereaved, through sharing fond memories, photos or videos. For young people who for practical or other reasons could not attend the funeral or visit the physical grave, the networking site became an online grave, a memorial place devoted to the lost friend. Sometimes sympathetic and personal messages were posted by strangers or peripheral friends who did not know the deceased very well. Although the majority of students positively evaluated the online experience of sharing grief and memorializing the deceased, for some was it like "confronting a ghost" ("It should be gone-he's gone. So, why is this still here?"; Hiefje, 2012; p. 37). Others felt uncomfortable and overwhelmed by new mementos, such as photos and videos, which were continually uploaded on the website.

Are online resources helpful in coping with loss and bereavement?

The bereaved who use online forums, chats, and email lists are mostly young adult women, less likely to be a part of a religious community, and the online resources are used quite frequently: the bereaved spend on the average approximately 7–8 hours online (Feigelman et al., 2008; van der Houwen et al., 2010b). Yet, despite an abundance of clinical and anecdotal evidence regarding the popularity of Internet use among the bereaved and the diversity of bereavement-related online activities and resources, there is not much evidence regarding their impact on the grief process and well-being of those who use them. Only a few methodologically sound studies, including controlled randomized trials, have been conducted, and these show effectiveness of professional online interventions such as Internet-based cognitive-behavioural therapy for complicated grief (Wagner, Knaevelsrud, & Maercker, 2006; 2007) and a brief Internet-based self-help intervention for the bereaved (van der

Houwen et al., 2010a). The majority of studies presented in the earlier parts of this chapter show high levels of satisfaction among members of online support groups, mailing lists, social networking sites, and individuals involved in online memorials. Still, such (mostly qualitative) studies suffer from problems plaguing research on Internet users, such as positive self-selection of participants (i.e., only people who are satisfied continue to use the websites and participate in research), lack of a comparison group, instability and changing membership of online groups, privacy issues and lack of follow-up (Eysenbach et al., 2004; Stroebe et al., 2008).

In general, bereavement literature suggests that involvement in online bereavement-related activities may be a valued addition to traditional bereavement activities as it creates connections with others who have suffered a loss and has a potential for enhancing a relationship with the deceased (Roberts, 2004). Indeed, studies show that the bereaved value the 24/7 availability, including weekends, holidays and anniversaries, of online forums and other sites (Swartwood et al., 2011). The online anonymity, often paired with an experience of social stigma and lack of direct social support, attract those who are trying to cope with disenfranchised grief or bereavement after suicide. For some people, expressing their feelings and thoughts writing online can be of therapeutic value (Lattanzi & Hale, 1984–1985; Roberts & Vidal, 2000). The bereaved used the Internet to find practical information, both on informative sites and through other bereaved, and to find support and understanding. Participants of online forums and social networking sites, as well as those involved in online memorials, evaluate positively their experience and report a sense of "online community" (Roberts, 2004). In addition, the Internet helps to maintain a continuing bond with the deceased through honouring his or her memory, tending the online grave and communicating with him or her via online messages (De Vries & Moldaw, 2012; Roberts, 2004).

On the other hand, concerns about possible dangers of seeking information and support via the Internet have been raised by both professionals and the bereaved (Chapple & Ziebland, 2011; Swartwood et al., 2011). Suicide survivors using the net, for instance, indicate that finding pro-suicide sites can be very distressing, and like other bereaved, they warn against treating the online activities as a substitute for (instead of supplement to) face-to-face contacts. Participation in a web forum or mailing list can become too time consuming or too depressing, and there is a risk of finding or offering unhelpful advice and/or misleading information. The impermanence of the Internet material, including online memorials, and changing membership in online groups can be a source of additional stress or loss. Concerns have also been raised about the "reluctance to let go" and the ruminative ways of grieving among some of the users and creators of such websites which may indicate poor adjustment (Stroebe et al., 2008). Last, but not least, dealing with the online legacy of the deceased, such as material left on a social networking site, might be experienced as facing an "online ghost" and may result in additional emotional and cognitive distress (Hiefje, 2012).

Ensuring quality of online information and support for the bereaved

A discussion of mental health resources available on the Internet, including bereavement-related material, inevitably leads to the questions regarding the quality of online information (Reavley & Jorm, 2011). Information provided on the Internet by professional organizations and services guarantees a high level of accuracy and recency of information, but such websites do not come up frequently in searches (Krysinska & Andriessen, 2010; Recupero et al., 2008). A number of initiatives have been implemented internationally to reduce the danger of misinformation when looking for (mental) health information online. These include MedCERTAIN, a European Union project aiming to establish a quality label for online health information (European Commission, 2002) and the Health On the Net Foundation (HON) Code (Health on the Net Foundation, 2012). The HONcode certificate is awarded to medical and health websites which meet the criteria of authority (information about authors' qualifications), complementarity (information supports, not replaces, contact with a health professional), confidentiality (respect for privacy of site users), attribution (citation of sources and dates), justifiability (presentation of justified, balanced and objective claims), transparency (valid authors' contact details), financial disclosure (details of funding) and advertising (advertising clearly distinguished from editorial content).

There are reports on development and qualitative evaluation of websites for the bereaved, including adolescent suicide survivors and their support networks in South Africa (Hoffmann, 2006) and the Internet-based psychoeducational tool "Making Sense of Grief" for the recently bereaved in the US (Dominick et al., 2009–2010). Also, quality criteria for health information have been recommended in the bereavement literature (Sofka, 2012b). Still, to-date there are no standard quality

Table 11.1 Recommended design for grief-related websites

Technical aspects	Design, colours and reading facility	Legal and ethical issues	Provision of emotional support	Resources, support organizations and other information
A home page with search facility	Minimalistic, simple design; no gimmicks, such as flowers or hearts	Provision of information, not advice	Welcoming paragraph*	Resources classified*, categorized under topic*, listed alphabetically by title rather than author*
A "how to use this site" page	Unobtrusive colours compatible with hope and conveying calm	Provision of quality information, including organizations and resources	Friendly language	A brief description of each book* and guidelines for ordering books/DVDs*
The side bar containing all functions	Consideration for colour blindness	A disclaimer and provision for professional indemnity and intellectual property	Direction to professional assistance	Support organizations listed by topic rather than geographically*
Contents and navigation instructions available at the top of each page	Maximum reading age of 8 years	Liability of a chat site	Chat site/links to chat sites/post it board	Non death-related loss information included*
No vertical columns with headings	Text in small blocks of print, dot points	Adherence to professional advertising conventions	Vignettes and quotes from real life stories*	
	Large, bold type fonts			

* Recommendations provided by the bereaved.

Source: Clark et al. (2004).

criteria for suicide bereavement websites, and the quality of available information differs (Krysinska & Andriessen, 2010).

One study which provides information about how to develop a quality and user-friendly bereavement website (http://grieflink.org.au) was conducted in Australia in collaboration with the bereaved by Clark and her colleagues (Clark et al., 2004). The authors stress the need to take into consideration the psychological needs of people who have experienced a recent loss. The grief process often impacts cognitive and emotional functioning, including concentration, memory and problem-solving. In the words of one of the bereaved, "(You) need to make it (the web site) very easy for bereaved people – its very difficult to think clearly and overcome obstacles" (Clark et al., 2004, p. 963). The bereaved can experience high levels of psychological distress and lowered self-esteem. Consequently, emotional support, such as a welcoming paragraph (e.g., "Welcome to GriefLink. We care about you."), should be provided on the home page, and the use of friendly and warm (not only informational) language is recommended. The information provided should be recent and accurate, and at the same time, easy to read, devoid of professional jargon and presented in small blocks of text, preferably with dot points. While mental health professionals and long-term bereaved value large amounts of information, the more recently bereaved prefer less information as "this is not a time when you can take much information in" (Clark et al., 2004, p. 966). Offering balanced, i.e., sufficient but not overwhelming, amount of information can be achieved by using links offering access to additional resources. Table 11.1 offers an overview of the recommendations provided by Clark and her colleagues (2004).

Conclusions

Based on material presented in this chapter, it can be unequivocally concluded that many suicide survivors and other bereaved use the Internet to seek information, to freely express their pain and to find others who have experienced a similar loss, and to memorialize and to connect to the deceased. Although more and more studies look at the frequency of Internet use in this group and its impact on the grief process, there remain many unanswered questions. The general suicide bereavement literature suggests that visiting and creating personal websites, such as Web memorials, may be a valued addition to traditional bereavement activities as it creates connections with others who have suffered a loss and has a potential for enhancing a relationship with the deceased (Roberts, 2004). We still lack scientific evidence to determine if creating or consulting suicide bereavement websites is a helpful addition to traditional bereavement activities, or if it hinders the grieving process through rumination and reluctance to let go. Also, the needs of individual survivors differ depending on their age, culture, gender and kinship relationship with the deceased (Andriessen, 2009; Jordan & McIntosh, 2011). One can ask if everyone finds online information and support suited to his/her individual needs?

Stroebe et al. (2008) observed that some Internet enthusiasts question the need to evaluate the efficacy of online support for the bereaved as long as the resources are provided for free, people use them voluntarily, and there is assurance that online information does not have adverse effects or is not misleading. However, they caution against accepting these assumptions without proper investigation. Indeed, development of quality standards and further research seem to be the next steps in providing online support for survivors after suicide.

References

Andriessen, K. (2009). Can postvention be prevention? *Crisis, 30*(1), 43–47.

Berger, M., Wagner, T. H., & Baker, L. C. (2005). Internet use and stigmatised illness. *Social Science and Medicine, 61*, 1821–1827.

Bocklandt, Ph. (ed.) (2011). *Niet alle smileys lachen. Onlinehulp in eerstelijnswelzijnswerk* [*Not all smileys are laughing. Online help in first line wellbeing services*]. Leuven/Den Haag: Acco.

Chapple, A., & Ziebland, S. (2011). How the Internet is changing the experience of bereavement by suicide: A qualitative study in the UK. *Health, 15*, 173–187.

Clark, S., Burgess, T., Laven, G., Bull, M., Marker, J., & Browne, E. (2004). Developing and evaluating the Grieflink web site: Processes, protocols, dilemmas and lessons learned. *Death Studies, 28*, 955–970.

Davison, K. P., Pennebaker, J. W., & Dickerson, S. S. (2000). Who talks? The social psychology of illness support groups. *American Psychologist, 55*, 205–217.

De Vries, B., & Moldaw, S. (2012). Virtual memorials and cyber funerals: Contemporary expressions of ageless experiences. In C. J. Sofka, I. Noppe Cupit & K. R. Gilbert (eds), *Dying, death, and grief in an online universe. For counselors and educators* (pp. 135–148). New York: Springer Publishing Company.

De Vries, B., & Rutherford, J. (2004). Memorializing loved ones on the World Wide Web. *Omega, 49*, 5–26.

Dominick, S. A., Irvine, A. B., Beauchamp, N., Seeley, J. R., Nolen-Hoeksema, S., Doka, K. J. & Bonanno, G. A. (2009–2010). An Internet tool to normalize grief. *Omega, 60*, 71–87.

European Commission (2002). MedPICS certification and rating of trustful and assessed health information on the net. Retrieved 30 June 2012, from http://ec.europa.eu/information_society/activities/sip/projects/completed/filtering_content_labelling/filtering/med_certain/index_en.htm.

Eysenbach, G., Powell, J., Englesakis, M., Rizo, C., & Stern, A. (2004). Health related virtual communities and electronic support groups: Systematic review of the effects of online peer to peer interactions. *British Medical Journal, 328,* 1166–1170.

Feigelman, W., Gorman, B. S., Beal, K. C., & Jordan, J. R. (2008). Internet support groups for suicide survivors: A new mode for gaining bereavement assistance. *Omega, 57,* 217–243.

Grad, O. (2011). The sequelae of suicide: Survivors. In R. C. O'Connor, S. Platt, & J. Gordon (eds), *International handbook of suicide prevention: Research, policy and practice* (pp. 561–575). New York: John Wiley & Sons.

Health on the Net Foundation (2012). Retrieved 30 June 2012, from http://www.hon.ch.

Health Service Executive (2011). Suicide prevention in the community: A practical guide. Retrieved 30 June 2012, from http://www.youthhealth.ie/sites/youthhealth.ie/files/Community%20Booklet%20Suicide-Prevention-1-March-2012.pdf.

Hiefje, K. (2012). The role of social networking sites in memorialization of college students. In C. J. Sofka, I. Noppe Cupit, & K. R. Gilbert (eds), *Dying, death, and grief in an online universe. For counselors and educators* (pp. 31–46). New York: Springer Publishing Company.

Hoffmann, W. A. (2006). Telematic technologies in mental health caring: A web-based psychoeducational program for adolescent suicide survivors. *Issues in Mental Health Nursing, 27,* 461–474.

Hollander, E. M. (2001). Cyber community in the valley of the shadow of death. *Journal of Loss and Trauma, 6,* 135–146.

Jordan, J. R., & McIntosh, J. L. (2011). Suicide bereavement: Why study survivors of suicide loss? In J. R. Jordan, & J. L. McIntosh (eds), *Grief after suicide* (pp. 3–17). New York: Routledge.

King, S. A., & Moreggi, D. (2007). Internet self-help and support groups: The pros and cons of text-based mutual aid. In J. Gackenbach (ed.), *Psychology and the Internet: Interpersonal, intrapersonal, and transpersonal implications.* (pp. 221–244). Boston: Academic Press.

Krysinska, K., & Andriessen, K. (2010). On-line support and resources for people bereaved through suicide: What is available? *Suicide & Life-threatening Behavior, 40,* 640–650.

Lattanzi, M., & Hale, M. E. (1984–1985). Giving grief words: Writing during bereavement. *Omega, 15,* 45–52.

Oliveri, T. (2003). Grief groups on the Internet. *Bereavement Care, 22,* 39–40.

Pew Research Center (2011). The social life of health information, 2011. Retrieved 30 June 2012, from http://pewinternet.org/Reports/2011/Social-Life-of-Health-Info.aspx.

Reavley, N. J., & Jorm, A. F. (2011). The quality of mental health information websites: A review. *Patient Education and Counseling, 85,* e16–e25.

Recupero, P. R., Harms, S. E., & Noble, J. M. (2008). Googling suicide: Surfing for suicide information on the internet. *Journal of Clinical Psychiatry, 69,* 878–888.

Roberts, P. (2004). The living and the dead: Community in the virtual cemetery. *Omega, 49,* 57–76.

Roberts, P., & Vidal, L. A. (2000). Perpetual care in cyberspace: A portrait of memorials on the Web. *Omega, 40,* 47–70.

Schalken, F., Wolters, W., Tilanus, W., van Gemert, M., van Hoogenhuyze, C. Meijer, E., ... Postel, M. (2010). *Handboek online hulpverlening. Hoe onpersoonlijk contact heel persoonlijk wordt* [*Handbook of online help. How impersonal contact becomes very personal*]. Houten: Bohn Stafleu van Loghum.

Socialbakers (2012). Facebook statistics by continents. Retrieved 30 June 2012, from http://www.socialbakers.com/countries/continents.

Sofka, C. J. (2012b). Informational support online: Evaluating resources. In C. J. Sofka, I. Noppe Cupit, & K. R. Gilbert (eds), *Dying, death, and grief in an online universe. For counselors and educators* (pp. 247–255). New York: Springer Publishing Company.

Stroebe, M. S., van der Houwen, K., & Schut, H. (2008). Bereavement support, intervention, and research on the Internet: A critical review. In M. S. Stroebe, R. O. Hanson, H. Schut, & W. Stroebe (eds), *Handbook of bereavement research and practice. Advances in theory and intervention* (pp. 551–554). Washington, DC: American Psychological Association.

Swartwood, R. M., McCarthy Veach, P., Kuhne, J., Lee, H. K., & Ji, K. (2011). Surviving grief: An analysis of the exchange of hope in online communities. *Omega, 63*, 161–181.

Tanis, M. (2007). Online social support groups. In A. Joinson, K. McKenna, T. Postmes, & U.-D. Reips (eds), *Oxford handbook of Internet psychology* (pp. 139–153). Oxford: Oxford University Press.

van der Houwen, K., Schut, H., van den Bout, J., Stroebe, M., & Stroebe, W. (2010a). The efficacy of a brief internet-based self-help intervention for the bereaved. *Behaviour Research and Therapy, 48*, 359–367.

van der Houwen, K., Stroebe, M., Schut, H., Stroebe, W., van den Bout, J. (2010b). Online mutual support in bereavement: An empirical investigation. *Computers in Human Behavior, 26*, 1519–1525.

Van Hecke, J. (ed.) (2012). *Internet als methodiek in de jeugdzorg. Een extra taal* [*Internet as a method in youth care. An extra language*]. Antwerpen: Garant.

Vanderwerker, L. C., & Prigerson, H. G. (2004). Social support and technological connectedness as protective factors in bereavement. *Journal of Loss and Trauma, 9*, 45–57

Wagner, B., Knaevelsrud, C., & Maercker, A. (2006). Internet-based cognitive-behavioral therapy for complicated grief: A randomized controlled trial. *Death Studies, 30*, 429–453.

Wagner, B., Knaevelsrud, C., & Maercker, A. (2007). Post-traumatic growth and optimism as outcomes of an Internet-based intervention for complicated grief. *Cognitive Behaviour Therapy, 36*, 156–161.

Williams, A. L., & Merten, M. J. (2009). Adolescents' online social networking following the death of a peer. *Journal of Adolescent Research, 24*, 67–90.

12

Innovating to Treat Depression and Prevent Suicide: The IPhone @PSY ASSISTANCE Application

Réal Labelle, Antoine Bibaud-De Serres and
François-Olivier Leblanc

Introduction

Smartphones may be on the verge of becoming a therapeutic adjunct and a useful adjunct to the treatment of depressed and suicidal persons. A Canadian research team has developed a mobile application for this client group. @Psy ASSISTANCE performs a variety of functions: it is a source of information, provides therapeutic support, collects data and serves as an emergency tool in the event of a crisis. The application's key function is its suicidal crisis safety plan. This six-part plan evaluates both the safety of the person's environment and warning signs of suicidal behaviour, and then suggests appropriate coping strategies. If distress levels demand rapid assistance, the instrument is programmed to make a call blast to five pre-determined individuals. In addition, the application geolocates the caller and nearby emergency care facilities. In the following sections, we present the background leading up to the development of the iPhone @Psy ASSISTANCE project and then describe the application and its utility.

Depression with or without suicidal behaviour

According to the World Health Organization, depression will become the second leading cause of disability worldwide by 2020 (World Health Organization, 2011) and the first in the industrialized countries by 2030 (Mathers & Loncar, 2006). In Canada, the lifetime prevalence rate of major depression is about 11 per cent for men and 16 per cent for women (Health Canada, 2009). Aside from the social impact in terms of human lives lost, the monetary costs related to depression and psychological distress have been estimated at about $14.4 billion per year in Canada (Stephens & Joubert, 2001).

Depression is also the psychopathology most associated with suicidal behaviour (Rihmer, Benazzi, & Gonda, 2007). From a conceptual point of view, suicidal behaviour is defined on a continuum from suicidal ideation to suicide attempts and completed suicides (Yufit & Lester, 2005). Suicidal ideation is the expression of a wish to die, which is generally considered serious when a detailed plan to kill oneself has been formulated. The degree of lethality of suicide attempts depends upon the means used and context. Although suicidal behaviour does not figure among the mental disorders of the DSM-IV-TR (American Psychiatric Association, 2000), it does constitute a symptom in the diagnoses of major depression (Axis I) and borderline personality disorder (Axis II). Oquendo, Baca-Garcia, and Giner (2008) recommended that suicidal behaviour be considered a separate diagnostic category documented on a sixth axis in the DSM-V.

Cognitive therapy for depression and suicide

Cognitive therapy has proved beneficial in treating depressed individuals with suicidal behaviour (Beck et al., 1979; Beck, 2011; Wenzel, Brown, & Beck, 2009). It is the intervention most validated for this purpose. According to two systematic reviews examining the results of 40 years of scientific research in the field (Beck, 2005; Butler et al., 2006), cognitive therapy is the preferred treatment for mild depression, an option in the treatment of moderate depression, and the treatment most indicated, in combination with antidepressants, in the case of severe depression with suicidal behaviour (American Psychiatric Association, 2010; Canadian Network for Mood and Anxiety Treatments, 2009; Institut national de santé et de la recherche médicale, 2004; Institut national de santé publique du Québec, 2012; National Institute for Health and Clinical Excellence, 2009).

Desktop computer-assisted cognitive therapy

The desktop computer has been used in various cognitive therapy programs in recent years. It has assisted users (therapists and patients) by offering a practical interface for therapeutic learning (Spurgeon & Wright, 2010). Beating the Blues (Proudfoot et al., 2003) and Good Days

Ahead (Wright, Wright, & Beck, 2002) are examples of programs where video exercises are part of the therapy. Control-group studies have demonstrated the effect of these interventions on diminishing mild and moderate depression in adults. (National Institute for Health and Clinical Excellence, 2006; Proudfoot et al., 2004).

Advent of mobile phone opens up new possibilities

Mobile phones seem well suited as an adjunct to cognitive therapy for depression and suicide. They make it possible to use applications anywhere at any time and to maintain contact with therapists between therapeutic sessions. Some researchers have been quick to recognize the utility of developing mobile applications in this field (Proudfoot et al., 2003; Proudfoot et al., 2004; Spek et al., 2007; Spurgeon & Wright, 2010; Wright et al., 2005).

According to the International Telecommunication Union (ITU), there were 5.9 billion mobile phone subscriptions globally in 2010. This translated into 78 subscriptions per 100 inhabitants worldwide (International Telecommunication Union, 2011). In the developed world, this proportion stood at 114.2, compared with 70.1 in the developing world (see Figure 12.1).

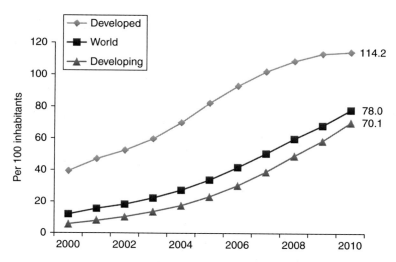

Figure 12.1   Mobile phone subscription rate for developed, developing and global world

Mobile telephony is unquestionably the fastest growing and most widespread of the various means of telecommunication. The above statistics might come as a surprise. However, it need be pointed out that the ITU is a United Nations agency whose purpose it is to document the evolution of telecommunications in its 152 member states. Each country's own statistics may vary in validity owing to disparities in resources available to national agencies. It is interesting to examine national averages in terms of subscriptions per inhabitant (International Telecommunication Union, 2011).

Mobile phones are interesting as instruments for psychotherapeutic intervention for several reasons. First, they can be purchased and maintained cheaply. Second, small and light, they can be easily carried in one's pants pockets or in a handbag. Finally, they can be relied upon to transmit messages, whether verbal (calls) or written (text messages), from just about anywhere. Thus, mobile phones can be used as therapeutic adjuncts to different ends, including telephone contact between sessions (Boschen & Casey, 2008). In addition, text messaging makes it possible to reach a vast number of patients automatically. This function has already been used, for example, to remind patients of aftercare services following certain medical treatments (Bauer et al., 2003; Franklin et al., 2006; Logan et al., 2007; Ryan et al., 2005).

In this regard, Chen, Mishara, and Liu (2010) set up a text-messaging program to follow up on 15 persons who visited an emergency clinic in China after attempting suicide. The messages sent provided support and a telephone contact in the event of a suicidal crisis. This pilot study showed that the use of test messages was a fast and inexpensive way to provide follow-up care in cases where aftercare is difficult to ensure.

Utility of smartphones in clinical practice and research

In recent years, a new generation of mobile phones has seen the light of day: smartphones. These combine the strengths of the computer and the mobile phone (Bang et al., 2007). Compared with their predecessors, smartphones offer two main advantages. First, these instruments function on higher performance telecommunication networks, such as the 3G network. Access to these networks allows transmitting data and surfing the internet independently of Wi-Fi networks, which require the user to be within reach of a router and modem. Among other things, this makes it easier and simpler for marginalized populations to use the smartphone's interface (Preziosa et al., 2009).

The second advantage offered by this technology is that it allows accessing multiple applications using a touch screen or a voice command, thus opening up new possibilities for clinical practice and research. Therapists and patients can now deposit and consult an impressive amount of information by using practical applications anywhere they want (Boschen, 2009). For researchers, smartphones are exceptional instruments for collecting data in real time and saving them directly on a server (Collins, Kashdan, & Gollnisch, 2003).

Examples of smartphone use in physical and psychological health

Medical settings around the world already use smartphones, particularly the iPhone, in their operations. They are employed, for example, as diagnostic aids (Dala-Ali, Lloyd, & Al-Abed, 2010), support for physiological measures (Joundi et al., 2011), schedule managers (Franklin et al., 2006; Logan et al., 2007; Ryan et al., 2005), support for consulting databases such as scientific reference libraries (Cuddy, 2008) and learning resource aids (Trelease, 2008).

In Canada, this new technology is presently being used at Mount Sinai Hospital in Toronto, where iPhones serve as a clinical data management tool and help optimize communication among professionals (Apple Inc., 2011). This project is based on the VitalHub application, an integrated health services system that connects all of the hospital's physicians via iPhone. This healthcare structure allows clinicians to consult and modify records on their mobile phones in real time with the utmost security. Furthermore, these instruments support immediate access to emails, diagnostic applications, contacts and the calendars of each member of the medical team. These are but a few examples of the promising possibilities that smartphones have opened up in other areas of healthcare.

Morris and colleagues (2010) developed a mobile application for assessing mood and proposing interventions through smartphones. To assess mood, the user responds to a series of questions regarding sadness and energy level, among other things. A random temporal pattern of follow-up calls is programmed to avoid habituation. Once the assessment is complete, exercises are proposed. These involve relaxation and cognitive re-evaluation. These authors reported a high degree of satisfaction with the application among the ten adult users they evaluated.

Rizvi, Dimeff, Skutch, Carroll, and Linehan (2011) developed and evaluated a smartphone application to support dialectical behaviour therapy interventions. The DBT Coach application is intended to enhance the generalization of a psychosocial skill, namely, opposite action (Linehan, 1993). More specifically, this application registers emotional measures and assesses how useful the application of this skill might be in a given situation. Measures of satisfaction and symptoms are gathered by both users and therapists. Results have shown use of DBT Coach to be associated with diminished depressive symptomatology and emotional intensity (Rizvi et al., 2011).

More recently, Wittaker and colleagues (2012) developed and tested an application intended to prevent depression among young people living in the community. MEMO automatically sends messages derived from cognitive-behavioural therapy (CBT) for depression. A total of 835 adolescents 13–17 years old participated in this efficacy study that compared the intervention group against a control group of adolescents who received messages on other subjects at the same rate. They found that more than 75 per cent of the adolescents read half of the messages and that 90.7 per cent of the intervention group would recommend the application to a friend. The adolescents who received messages derived from CBT reported that the application helped them to be more positive and to get rid of negative thoughts more easily, compared with the control group.

To our knowledge, there exists no prior smartphone application for treating both depression and suicide based on cognitive therapy. An automated search on Apple's iTune Store run in January 2013 on the words depression, suicide, cognitive therapy, behaviour therapy and their French equivalents did turn up a hundred or so iPhone applications. These included applications on: (i) various self-treatment interventions, (ii) diagnostic impressions and screening, (iii) mood self-assessment, (iv) suicidal crisis emergency assistance, (v) psycho-education for service users, (vi) treatment guidelines for therapists and (vii) various social support networks. In light of the articles and applications reviewed, it appeared relevant to develop a unifying, personalized and interactive smartphone application that could serve as an adjunct to cognitive therapy for depression with or without suicidal complications.

A novel multifunction iPhone application for depressed and suicidal persons

In the aim of making the most of cognitive therapy, Labelle and Bibaud-De Serres (2012) developed an original multifunctional application for depressed and suicidal persons: @Psy ASSISTANCE. This application is at the same time a documentary resource, a therapeutic tool, a data collector and a source for emergency help in the event of a crisis. Intended as an extension of the therapeutic relation, it is accessible 24/7 thanks to advances in technology. Furthermore, @Psy ASSISTANCE is designed in such a way that if the level of distress necessitates rapid support, the instrument is programmed to make what is known as a "call blast." When this occurs, five persons with whom an agreement has been established beforehand are contacted. The first two persons reached are automatically placed in a conference call with the depressed and suicidal person. A geolocalization function also allows quickly determining the person's whereabouts. If the situation requires it, the application is ready to immediately contact a therapist, crisis centre, the nearest hospital or 911. The quickest route to the designated facility can be displayed on the screen. As a result, individuals are able to obtain appropriate help easily and as quickly as possible.

The application's three objectives are to inform, empower and protect. First, @Psy ASSISTANCE informs by allowing users to consult educational video clips, recommended readings, a list of resources, and selected and personalized hyperlinks. Second, it empowers users by allowing them to do clinical exercises specially selected for them, such as behavioural

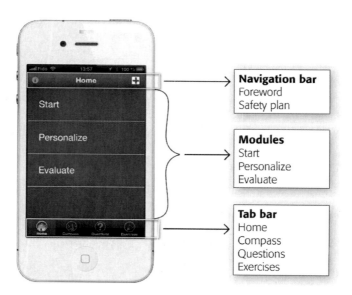

Figure 12.2A   Example of @Psy ASSISTANCE screenshots

activation, problem solving and cognitive restructuring. It further empowers them by making it possible to gather data from observations of their mood in real time and to consult their clinician's latest recommendations in a wide variety of forms (images, tables, charts, audio and video messages, questionnaires), all of this through an interactive platform that allows information to be exchanged between patients and therapists. Finally, and this is clearly the most revolutionary aspect of the application, it protects vulnerable users by including among its functions an emergency plan available at one's fingertip in the event of a suicidal crisis. Divided into six steps, the plan assesses the security of the user's environment and warning signs of suicidal behaviour, proposes immediate coping strategies and deploys a series of rescue

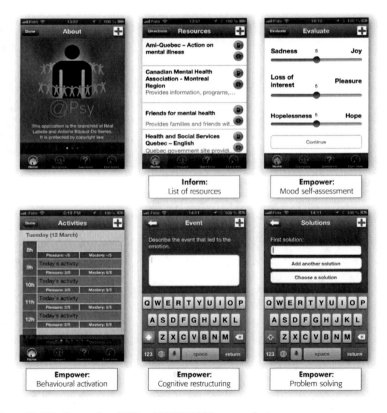

Figure 12.2B Example of @Psy ASSISTANCE screenshots

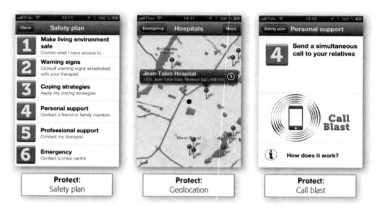

Figure 12.2C   Example of @Psy ASSISTANCE screenshots

actions graduated on the basis of distress level. Figures 12.2A, 12.2B and 12.2C provide examples of the application's functions.

Development stages of @Psy ASSISTANCE mobile application

The application's development went through three distinct stages, in accordance with the Canadian Innovation Commercialization Program (Government of Canada, 2012). First, a preliminary version was produced. At this stage, researchers implemented the concept of the application. The research team defined the application's domain, determined its relevance, examined existing therapeutic protocols and reviewed existing applications.

More specifically, it was established that the instrument in question fell within the domain of mental health care and smartphones. Next, with the goal of defining its utility, the research team identified needs in psychotherapy and possibilities afforded by new technologies. The concept of the application was born at the juncture of these two spheres, that is, the idea of exploiting the qualities of the iPhone (portability, interactivity, flexibility) to meet the need to inform, empower and protect patients more effectively. Then, the cognitive therapy protocol for depressed patients (Beck et al., 1979; Beck, 2011) and the cognitive therapy protocol for suicidal patients (Wenzel, Brown, & Beck, 2009) were selected for their relevance. The different modules proposed by the authors of these protocols were identified, and their usefulness for the smartphone application was evaluated. The modules deemed most relevant were selected, and a process of reflection was undertaken on the application's technical aspects. It should be noted that, in conducting this process, consideration was given to the recommendations made by Williams and Whitfield (2001) concerning the adaptation of traditional therapeutic material to a novel technological environment. Following those guidelines, the emphasis was placed on: 1) accessibility, by simplifying the design and layout; 2) appropriateness, by ensuring the material was designed for suicidal and depressive users; 3) legibility, by verifying that the content was clearly presented while keeping the medico-technical language to a minimum; and 4) user involvement, by involving users and therapists in the development, validation and evaluation process. A review of existing applications was carried out to confirm the project's innovative dimension.

In the second stage of development, a preliminary version of the application was produced. This involved the process of programming the application's different modules. The aim here was for the programmer to appropriate the basic concepts of cognitive therapy and for the psychologists to appropriate the iPhone environment. Then, the psychotherapeutic concepts were operationalized in computer terms. This meant translating and adapting the different modules for use on a small screen. Large tables normally used on paper were fractioned and divided into numerous screens accessible by touching buttons or scrolling. The next step was to program the components. For this preliminary version, it was decided that the native application would comprise six sections. First, the Safety plan evaluates both the safety of a person's environment and warning signs of suicidal behaviour, and then suggests appropriate coping strategies, starting with personalized ones, to relieve the stress felt. The Safety plan is designed to allow the user to adjust the emergency level to the situation. If distress levels demand rapid assistance, the instrument is programmed to make a call blast to five pre-determined individuals, who are then connected to the user on a conference call. The user is also invited to call healthcare professionals involved in his treatment by using pre-registered numbers. If these steps are not indicated for the situation, the application can geolocate the caller and identify emergency care facilities, call a suicide hotline or allow the user to call 911 automatically as a last resort. Second, the Home section covers personalization settings, which allow choosing a data privacy code and modifying phone numbers for the safety plan, and therapist settings for data exchange with the server. The Home section also includes a daily mood self-evaluation with graphs to monitor fluctuations and tutorials describing and demonstrating the application's functions . Third, the Compass section covers treatment information, relapse prevention, useful resources reachable by phone or the web, and recommended readings embedded in the application. Fourth, the Questions section offers psycho-educational video clips on depression, its treatment and relevant bits of advice to foster recovery. Information is presented in a comprehensible manner. Fifth, the Exercises section covers three common modules in cognitive therapy: behavioural activation, cognitive restructuration and problem solving. These exercises are usually explained by the therapist and serve to help the user put into practice the skills learned in psychotherapy. Sixth and last, the About section presents legal information on property rights.

This stage also entailed determining the relationship between a secured remote server, the web portal and the iPhone application. This is because the @Psy ASSISTANCE application is programmed to send and receive user data to and from a distant server and the therapist is allowed to access it by consulting the server via a web page.

In the third stage, an experimental version of the application was produced. A committee of experts was formed in the summer of 2011 including three university professors of psychology (and members of the Order of Psychologists of Quebec), a doctoral student, and a software engineering student. The committee obtained the viewpoints of specialists in order to make necessary changes to the application. More than a dozen versions were produced by the engineer and corrected by the development team. Aside from the application itself, several documents were produced as well: (1) a user's guide for patients, (2) a user's guide for therapists, and (3) a provisional patent at the United States Trademark and Patent Office.

How the @Psy ASSISTANCE application contributes to cognitive therapy for depression and suicide

First, the @Psy ASSISTANCE application centralizes and provides access to all of the therapeutic components recommended in cognitive therapy through technological means. For example, being able to access in a few seconds a series of psycho-educational video clips, relevant resources, mood self-assessments and personalized reading material allows therapists to deliver in an innovative manner the tasks that need to be accomplished in the course of psychotherapy for depression. Patients affected by depression, whose motivation is typically diminished, benefit in particular from seeing their therapeutic environment synthesized in a single application they can carry around with them and access anytime.

For suicide prevention, the application's principal appeal lies in one particular module: the Suicidal Crisis Safety Plan. A suicidal crisis can be described as a state of insufficiency in terms of coping mechanisms. A safety plan could be useful in this context by reminding patients to apply their own coping mechanisms judiciously in order to prevent a crisis. What the technology adds in particular to the safety plan is an automatic call function. This allows individuals experiencing different levels of distress to easily reach their external resources, including friends, family, and mental health professionals.

Conclusion

In sum, depression with or without suicidal behaviour is a major public health concern. The cognitive therapy protocols developed by Aaron Beck (Beck, 2005; Beck et al., 1979; Beck, 2011) and Wenzel et al. (2009) are interventions developed to treat depressed patients with or without suicidal behaviour. These interventions are among some of the most scientifically validated treatments available today. Recent research has emphasized both the importance of doing exercises at home and the suicidal crisis safety plan as ways of boosting the effectiveness of cognitive therapy with depressed and suicidal patients and helping to prevent a suicide attempt. Recent studies have examined the use of computers in self-treatment and therapeutic assistance programs. A review of programs presently available revealed that this type of intervention has been reserved for patients with subclinical symptom levels and no suicidal behaviour. Moreover, although they are more interactive, desktop computers present various limitations, especially with respect to portability. From this perspective, the proliferation of mobile phones, and even more so of smartphones, opens up the promising possibility of using them as therapeutic adjuncts to cognitive therapy for depressed and suicidal patients. The development of a mobile application called @ Psy ASSISTANCE meets this need by providing a technological means to treat depression and prevent suicide more effectively.

References

American Psychiatric Association. (2000). *Diagnostic and statistical manual of mental disorders* (4th ed., text rev.). Washington, DC: Author.

American Psychiatric Association. (2010). *Practice guideline for the treatment of patients with major depressive disorder* (3rd ed.). Washington, DC: Author.

Apple Inc. (2011). Mount Sinai Hospital: iPhone provides the vital link to medical records. Retrieved from: http://www.apple.com/iphone/business/profiles/mt-sinai/

Bang, M., Timpka, T., Eriksson, H., Holm, E., & Nordin, C. (2007). Mobile phone computing for in-situ cognitive behavioral therapy. *Studies in Health Technology and Informatics, 129*, 1078–1082.

Bauer, S., Percevic, R., Okon, E., Meermann, R., & Kordym, H. (2003). Use of text messaging in the aftercare of patients with bulimia nervosa. *European Eating Disorders Review, 11*(3), 279–290.

Beck, A. T. (2005). The current state of cognitive therapy: A 40-year retrospective. *Archives of General Psychiatry, 62*(2), 953–959.

Beck, A. T., Rush, A. J., Shaw, B. F., & Emery, G. (1979). *Cognitive therapy of depression*. New York, NY: Guilford Press.

Beck, J. S. (2011). *Cognitive behavior therapy: Basics and beyond* (2nd ed.). New York, NY: Guilford Press.

Boschen, M. J. (2009). Mobile telephones and psychotherapy: I. Capability and applicability. The Behavior Therapist, 32(8), 168–175.

Boschen, M. J., & Casey, L. M. (2008). The use of mobile telephones as adjuncts to cognitive behavioral psychotherapy. *Professional Psychology: Research and Practice, 39*(5), 546–552.

Butler, A. C., Chapman, J. E., Forman, E. M., & Beck, A. T. (2006). The empirical status of cognitive-behavioral therapy: A review of meta-analyses. *Clinical Psychology Review, 26*(1), 17–31.

Canadian Network for Mood and Anxiety Treatments. (2009). Clinical guidelines for the management of major depressive disorder in adults. *Journal of Affective Disorders, 117*(1), S1–S64.

Chen, H., Mishara, B. L., & Liu, X. X. (2010). A pilot study of mobile telephone message interventions with suicide attempters in China. *Crisis, 31*(2), 109–112.

Collins, R. L., Kashdan, T. B., & Gollnisch, G. (2003). The feasibility of using cellular phones to collect ecological momentary assessment data: Application to alcohol consumption. *Experimental and Clinical Psychopharmacology, 11*(1), 73–78.

Cuddy, C. (2008). The iPhone in medical libraries. *Journal of Electronic Resources in Medical Libraries, 5*(3), 287–292.

Dala-Ali, B. M., Lloyd, A. L., & Al-Abed, Y. (2010). The uses of the iPhone for surgeons. *The Surgeon, 9*(1), 44–48.

Franklin, V. L., Waller, A., Pagliari, C., & Greene, S. A. (2006). A randomized controlled trial of sweet talk, a text messaging system to support young people with diabetes. *Diabetic Medicine, 23*(12), 1332–1338.

Government of Canada (2012). Technology readiness levels. Retrieved from: https://buyandsell.gc.ca/initiatives-and-programs/canadian-innovation-commercialization-program-cicp/program-specifics/technology-readiness-levels

Health Canada. (2009). It's your health. Mental health – depression. Retrieved from: http://www.hc-sc.gc.ca

Institut national de santé et de la recherche médicale. (2004). *Psychothérapie : Trois approches évaluées [Psychotherapy: Three approaches evaluated]*. Paris, France: Author.

Institut national de santé publique du Québec. (2012). *Faire face à la dépression au Québec – Protocole de soins à l'intention des intervenants de première ligne [Dealing with depression in Quebec: Care protocol for frontline service providers]*. Montreal, Canada: Centre de recherche du CHUM.

International Telecommunication Union. (2011). *Measuring the information society: The ICT Development Index 2011*. Geneva, Switzerland: Author.

Joundi, R. A., Brittain, J. S., Jenkinson, N., Green, A. L., & Aziz, T. (2011). Rapid tremor frequency assessment with the iPhone accelerometer. *Parkinsonism and Related Disorders, 17*(4), 288–290.

Labelle, R., & Bibaud-De Serres, A. (2012). *U.S. provisional patent no. 288.156.7*. Washington, DC: U.S. Patent and Trademark Office.

Linehan, M. M. (1993). *Cognitive-behavioral treatment of borderline personality disorder*. New York, NY: Guilford Press.

Logan, A. G., McIsaac, W. J., Tisler, A., Irvine, M. J., Saunders, A., Dunai, A., … Cafazzo, J. A. (2007). A mobile phone based remote patient monitoring system for management of hypertension in diabetic patients. *American Journal of Hypertension, 20*(9), 942–948.

Mathers, C. D., & Loncar, D. (2006). Projections of global mortality and burden of disease from 2002 to 2030. *PLoS Medicine, 3*(11), 2011–2030.

Morris, M. E., Kathawala, Q., Leen, T. K., Gorenstein, E. E., Guilak, F., Labhard, M., & Deleeuw, W. (2010). Mobile therapy: Case study evaluations of a cell phone application for emotional self-awareness. *Journal of Medical Internet Research, 12*(2), e10.

National Institute for Health and Clinical Excellence. (2006). *Computerised cognitive behaviour therapy for depression and anxiety. Clinical guideline no. 51*. London, UK: Author.

National Institute for Health and Clinical Excellence. (2009). *Depression treatment and management of depression in adults, including adults with a chronic physical health problem. Quick reference guide*. London, UK: Author.

Oquendo, M.A., Baca-Garcia, E., & Giner, J. (2008). Issues for DSM-V: Suicidal behavior as a separate diagnosis on a separate axis. *American Journal of Psychiatry, 165*, 1383–1384.

Preziosa, A., Grassi, A., Gaggioli, A., & Riva, G. (2009). Therapeutic applications of the mobile phone. *British Journal of Guidance and Counselling, 37*(3), 313–325.

Proudfoot, J., Goldberg, D., Mann, A., Everitt, B., Marks, I., & Gray, J. A. (2003). Computerized, interactive, multimedia cognitive-behavioural therapy reduces anxiety and depression in general practice: A randomized controlled trial. *Psychological Medicine, 33*(2), 217–227.

Proudfoot, J., Ryden, C., Everitt, B., Shapiro, D. A., Goldberg, D., Mann, A., … Gray, J.A. (2004). Clinical efficacy of computerised cognitive-behavioural therapy for anxiety and depression in primary care: Randomised controlled trial. *British Journal of Psychiatry, 185*, 46–54.

Rihmer, Z., Benazzi, F., & Gonda, X. (2007). Suicidal behavior in unipolar depression: Focus on mixed states. In R. Tartarelli, M. Pompili, & P. Girardi (eds), *Suicide in psychiatric disorders* (pp. 101–113). New York, NY: Nova Science Publishers.

Rizvi, S. L., Dimeff, L. A., Skutch, J., Carroll, D., & Linehan, M. M. (2011). A pilot study of the DBT Coach: An interactive mobile phone application for individuals with borderline personality disorder and substance use disorder. *Behavior Therapy, 42*(4), 589–600.

Ryan, D., Cobern, W., Wheeler, J., Price, D., & Tarassenko, L. (2005). Mobile phone technology in the management of asthma. *Journal of Telemedicine and Telecare, 11*(Suppl. 1), 43–46.

Spek, V., Cuijpers, P., Nykliček, I., Riper, H., Keyzer, J., & Pop, V. (2007). Internet-based cognitive behaviour therapy for symptoms of depression and anxiety: A meta-analysis. *Psychological Medicine, 37*(3), 319–328.

Spurgeon, J. A., & Wright, J. H. (2010). Computer-assisted cognitive-behavioral therapy. *Current Psychiatry Reports, 12*(6), 547–552.

Stephens, T., & Joubert, N. (2001). Le fardeau économique des problèmes de santé mentale au Canada [The economic burden of mental health problems in Canada]. *Maladies chroniques au Canada, 22*(1), 18–23.

Trelease, R. B. (2008). Diffusion of innovations: Smartphones and wireless anatomy learning resources. *Anatomical Sciences Education, 1*(6), 233–239.

Wenzel, A., Brown, G., & Beck, A. T. (2009). *Cognitive therapy for suicidal patients: Scientific and clinical applications.* Washington, DC: American Psychological Association.

Williams, C. J., & Whitfield, G. (2001). Written and computer-based self-help treatments for depression. *British Medical Bulletin, 57*(1), 133–144.

Wittaker, R., Merry, S., Stasiak, K., McDowell, H., Doherty, I., Shepherd, M., & Dorey, E. (2012). MEMO-A mobile phone depression prevention intervention for adolescents: Development process and post-program findings on acceptability from a randomized controlled trial. *Journal of Medical Internet Research, 14*(1), e13.

World Health Organization. (2011). Depression. Retrieved from: http://www. who.int/mental_health/management/depression/definition /en/#

Wright, J. H., Wright, A. M., Albano, A. M., Basco, M. R., Goldsmith, J. L., Raffield, T., & Otto, M. W. (2005). Computer-assisted cognitive therapy for depression: Maintaining efficacy while reducing therapist time. *American Journal of Psychiatry, 162*, 1158–1164.

Wright, J. H., Wright, A. S., & Beck, A. T. (2002). *Good days ahead: The multimedia program for cognitive therapy.* Louisville, KY: Mindstreet.

Yufit, R. I., & Lester, D. (2005). *Assessment, treatment, and prevention of suicidal behavior.* Hoboken, NJ: John Wiley.

13
Promising Practices, Future Prospects and Research Agenda

Ad J. F. M. Kerkhof and Brian L. Mishara

We are currently witnessing a rapid growth of independent initiatives using new technologies in suicide prevention, often unaware of each other's activities. Their objectives are quite diverse, including to: improve screening, provide self-diagnosis, increase awareness, offer mutual support, provide guided and unguided self-help, access crisis intervention by text messaging, ensure safety planning and much more. To date, there is no central forum, exchange or repository of the various initiatives and experiences. Suicidal individuals seeking help are at the mercy of search engines that identify sites by popularity, rather than their usefulness or appropriateness. In addition, each newly developed service or application is competing for "market share", and few of the technological innovations are freely shared with others. It would be useful for a worldwide organization to provide a portal for accessing all reliable sources of information and help, as well as to develop a platform for sharing information in order to facilitate advancement in the field.

As is usually the case when new prevention measures are tried, research is lagging behind in evaluating the effects of these new technologies. This means that we do not yet know which of these initiatives work most effectively, under what conditions and whether they really help prevent suicides. In this final chapter, we suggest which developments seem promising to pursue, we examine potential pitfalls in developing new technologically supported interventions and we suggest a priority research agenda for the future.

Suicidal people increasingly surf the Internet for information about how to commit suicide, and they can easily find the many websites that offer explicit descriptions of suicide methods. Just type in Google: *how to commit suicide?* You will find a lot of nonsense, sick humour, as well as explicit, not always reliable, information about the pros and cons of particular methods, including their speed, reliability and likely amount of pain associated with each. There are pro-suicide websites that encourage or glorify suicide, similar to websites that promote anorexia (pro-ana). In Belgium and the Netherlands banners appear warning every visitor of pro-ana websites (*You are now on the point of entering a website with unhealthy and dangerous advice. Do not follow this advice, but instead click here to go to an objective website on anorexia*). Similar initiatives are being developed to warn visitors who are at the point of entering a pro-suicide website. However, there are important ethical and practical concerns whenever there is an attempt to categorize or label a site as dangerous or unhealthy. New web sites appear constantly and it requires extensive resources to constantly monitor all sites on a topic and make valid decisions about their dangers. At the present time auto-mated monitoring programmes are far from perfect. A programme set to label sites that provide information about suicide methods risks to warn Internet users of the dangers of entering suicide prevention sites, such as the World Health Organization or the International Association for Suicide Prevention sites because of their discussions on the prevention of the use of various methods. In addition, they may miss identifying "dangerous" sites that do not use the key words and phrases that the programme identifies as being dangerous.

Social media messages with suicidal content are regularly being read by "friends," without anyone intervening. In several countries, including Belgium, the Centres for the Prevention of Suicide and Facebook collab-orate to stimulate people who read a suicidal message to use a report button connecting the sender to a banner from the centre to help him deal with the suicidal communication.

In the e-mental health field many studies have demonstrated the effectiveness of guided or unguided web-based self- help for mental disorders, such as depression, panic disorder, general anxiety disorder, social phobia and problem drinking. Recently a study of an Internet Cognitive Behavioural Therapy (CBT) intervention for depression showed a decrease in suicidal ideation (Watts et al., 2012). Such devel-opments should now be implemented and studied with the treatment of suicidal patients.

People have their smartphones with them all day long. This means that a smartphone can become a 24-hour buddy every day, that at any suitable moment can remind you of agreements you made with your psychotherapist, can initiate an intervention when your sadness levels drop dangerously, and who stays with you to provide support and can help you communicate to obtain support when everyone else has left you. You may even create your own smartphone avatar buddy to help you do sensible things in times of crisis. One of the authors (AK) is now developing smartphone applications for safety plans for suicidal outpatients and for those who leave the general hospital after attempted suicide. Stanley and Brown (2012) developed a brief intervention to mitigate suicide risk by preparing safety plans for patients after attempted suicide before they leave the hospital emergency room. It would be interesting to see how this might be transferred into a smartphone application. As we have seen in Chapter 12 by Labelle and colleagues, it is also possible to develop computer programs which monitor in a smartphone how people are doing and automatically sends out a call for help to several members of the person's support network should a suicidal crisis develop. In Sri Lanka, a brief mobile phone treatment intervention after attempted suicide revealed promising results. The intervention included training in problem-solving therapy and meditation, a brief intervention to increase social support as well as advice on alcohol and drugs and mobile phone follow-up (Marasinghe et al., 2012).

Issues of sufficient helpers and repeated users

At the present time, most new technologies used in suicide prevention involve trained professionals or volunteers using the Internet or other technologies as a tool in helping suicidal individuals. This may involve self-testing, engaging with individuals in a chat, sending text messages to follow-up with a suicide attempter or entering a discussion forum to dissuade someone from proceeding with their suicide plans.

There are common pitfalls for these lifeline services. It takes a huge number of volunteers and professionals to guarantee 7-days-a-week, 24-hour access. The demand for telephone and chat services is unevenly distributed during the day, and at some "peak" periods suicidal persons may need to be put on hold and have to wait considerably before a helper is available. At other times, for example during the early morning hours, the demand is usually low and it is sometimes difficult to find workers for these shifts.

Another serious pitfall is that a considerable percentage of all chats and telephone calls concern a rather small number of persons who very frequently access the telephone or chat service. Some visitors use the chat or telephone hundreds of times a month, and thus tend to obstruct the access for other users. It may be that this small number of callers and chatters develop a suicidal identity and look for continuous help without any indication of change or effect. This is a serious problem for many services, and some services attempt a form of pre-selection or triage before callers or chatters are being put through to a volunteer. However, unlike telephone helplines that have the possible advantage of recognition of a person's voice, it is not easy to identify frequent users of Internet services, when the contact is by written text and from users who may change servers, camouflage IP numbers and use different identities.

A further problem for these services is that it is often difficult for workers to refer callers and chatters to later professional treatment if needed. Often chatters and callers have had negative experiences with mental health care, and they do not want to be referred to these services again. Or because of shame, or feelings of being an intractable case, or fear of stigma, or for whatever reason, they are difficult to be motivated to enter subsequent off-line regular mental health care treatment. Still it remains important to motivate callers and chatters to try regular treatment. Problems with making referrals are further exacerbated when the caller is in another country or geographic region where the service provider is not aware of local resources.

Because of these pitfalls, it is important for hotline services to conduct research into the effectiveness of their work in terms of providing emotional support, crisis intervention, and persuading and motivating suicidal callers and chatters to regular mental health care. It is also important to research the different characteristics of suicidal callers and chatters and particularly extremely repetitive callers and chatters.

Who is willing to pay for help over the Internet?

When telephone helplines began, callers almost invariably came from the area where the service was established, and the local community that was served provided funding for the services. With the advent of cheap long-distance and national toll free numbers, many countries and areas now provide a network of helplines that each share a proportion of the calls, with priority routing of calls to the centre in the region from which the call originated. The use of local centres is often justified by the fact that local knowledge is useful in order to identify resources, for example emergency services to send in the case of a suicide attempt and local mental health services where someone can be referred for long term help. However, the Internet knows no borders. Attempts to screen users of services based on ISP addresses are quite difficult and often inaccurate. Therefore, there are issues of who is paying to help whom. For example, when one city in Quebec, Canada, funded the local suicide prevention centre to offer help over the Internet, they were soon surprised to learn that the majority of users of the service were from outside their region, despite careful attempts at limiting publicity about the service to the local area. Funders tend to be territorial, and in the case of the Quebec initiative, the local funders refused to continue to finance the expanding service because the majority of clients were not taxpayers from their region.

One of the biggest challenges for the future of Internet-based help is to determine who will be providing the services and who will be financing them. One solution is to pool resources by offering services through a single regional, national or international common portal. However, most health and mental health services, including suicide prevention, are funded by a specific jurisdiction to serve the residents of that jurisdiction. This may be less of an issue when the language in which the services are provided does not cross borders and the funder is a federal government or national charity that represents most people who speak that language. However, when services are provided in a language that is shared by several countries, such as English, French or Arabic, there are the ethical, practical and financial issues of either accepting or trying to screen out service users who are outside the area funding the services.

"Push" versus "Pull" prevention technologies and their ethical and practical challenges

At the present time almost all Internet-based suicide prevention activities use "pull" technologies, that is, the services are available and users must actively go to, find or initiate contact with potential sources of help. It is also possible to develop proactive interventions using "push" technologies where one actively seeks out people who may potentially be suicidal and then offer help or try to dissuade a person at risk from proceeding with a suicide attempt. In the case of push technologies, the suicidal person does not overtly ask for help, but help is offered or provided regardless. It is both an ethical and practical issue to determine whether one should actively scan the Internet or certain Internet activities and initiate unsolicited contacts to try to prevent suicides. Then, there is the as yet unexplored evaluation research issue of whether or not such efforts actually do prevent suicides.

At the present time, one of the authors (BLM) has been categorizing the behaviours of people who commit suicide in the Montreal Metro (subway) System by analysing videotapes of their behaviour from the time they enter the station until their suicide. He is examining the potential of identifying behavioural patterns that would signal to surveillance personnel watching television monitors to pay attention to a specific individual in a specific station. One of the challenges to having thousands of television monitors in a public transit system is that there are not enough people to accurately look at all of them all the time. However a computer program could analyse simultaneously all the television monitors in all the stations and, if they can identify patterns of human behaviour which may be indicative of a potential suicide attempt, they can signal people monitoring the TVs to have a look and see if they might want to slow down the train coming into that station or send someone to see if there is a need to intervene with a suicidal individual.

Obviously, this may seem like Big Brother is watching, and some people may become concerned about people observing their behaviour in public places and perhaps sometimes intervening when they have not broken any laws and no intervention is warranted. However, there are both advantages and disadvantages concerning privacy issues when the monitoring being conducted by a computer rather than a human. The advantage is that the focus is only on specific behaviours that may indicate suicide risk and no person is observing any other behaviours which people might be embarrassed about, but are not indicative of any danger. The disadvantage is that there will be more false positives because the behavioural indicators of a potential suicide attempt are also indicators of people who are distraught or nervous. For example, someone who leaves a package and gets up and moves towards the tracks may be someone who is considering jumping and has left their possessions behind, but it could also be someone who is simply forgetful. Someone who seems very anxious and keeps looking over the edge towards the train may be anticipating a suicide or may be just very late for an important appointment. Again, there are important ethical issues about when some form of intervention is justified. If the only intervention is slowing the train before it comes into the station, that does not specifically impact the person who is observed. However, if the police arrive and start questioning the person, some people could be upset by a needless intervention, even though some lives are sometimes saved.

Today, Internet users are bombarded by publicity which uses their Internet behaviours to target them for certain types of publicity and promotes sales of the specific products which people are more likely to use based upon where they have previously visited on the Internet. Thus, when someone browses used car announcements on Google and looks at Land Rovers for sale, various pop-up advertising for local Land Rover dealers will "happen" to appear in increasing frequencies. Similarly, programs can be designed to identify Internet users who might be likely candidates for receiving help because of their suicide risk. Perhaps they could receive pop-up windows with links to services in suicide prevention or, in extreme cases when it seems likely someone is about to commit suicide, a suicide prevention organization could initiate contact with the person without ever being asked to provide help.

There are obvious ethical issues in proactive interventions, when compared to helping people who seek help overtly. Mishara & Weisstub (2010) compared the ethical premises used by Samaritan organizations in the United Kingdom, which only accept to help people who seek them out and respect the decision of callers to decide for themselves to live or die, with the position of United-States helplines affiliated with the National Suicide Prevention Lifeline Network (NSPL). NSPL member centres are obliged to trace calls (and if possible trace locations over the Internet for chat participants) and send emergency services if a suicide attempt is in progress or is imminent. In both countries, however, one can justify the intervention by the fact that the caller initiated an activity to obtain help from the organization since the caller intentionally contacted an organization whose mandate is to prevent suicides. It is a quite different situation when no explicit request for help or contact with a help-giving organization is made, but the person is identified as being at suicidal risk based on observed public behaviours over the Internet. Some say that this is the same as someone walking down the street and seeing someone ready to jump off a bridge. However, the difference is that the computer searching for people at risk of suicide is not a chance observer. It is not even comparable to having television surveillance cameras on a bridge, where the potential suicide victim is initiating actions to enter a location where television surveillance is known as being present. Hunting for potential suicide attempters in their public Internet activities is not as traumatic an intrusion into privacy as would be going into someone's home and looking to see if they are planning suicide. Over the Internet, we are observing behaviour that is public in the sense that it is open for anyone perusing the Internet to see. However, the proactive nature of actively seeking to identify someone as being at suicide risk poses unique ethical concerns about its potentially intrusive nature when there are no indications that the suicide victim wants anyone to help.

Using the arguments developed by Mishara and Weisstub (2005, 2007, 2010), we can justify proactively trying to identify potentially suicidal people on the Internet by a moralistic view that protection of life is more important than any potential intrusion into privacy. Furthermore, one could ask if public behaviour on the Internet does guarantee any form of privacy. If Google can send us advertising promoting a certain brand of car or a specific car dealership based on our Internet behaviour, shouldn't one be able to offer help for someone displaying Internet behaviours indicative of greater suicide risk? One could also use consequentialist arguments if one were to find, as is the case for telephone helplines, when they send ambulances against people's will, that people usually call back to thank the helpline for saving their lives. On the other hand, if one believes that people have a right to decide for themselves to commit suicide or not, any interventions could be seen as not warranted. However, even people with this belief in individual decision making may allow some form of "minimal" sharing of information. For example, this could be in the form of informing people at risk of suicide of the presence of a helpline, so that they may then choose for themselves to either use that help or not. For a greater discussion of these ethical issues see Mishara and Weisstub (2005, 2007, 2010), and Chapter 5 in this book.

Automated interventions

In the early 1970s we saw the development of computer programs which mimicked Rogerian non-directive psychotherapy. The software program called Eliza, developed by Joseph Weizenbaum, a professor at the Massachusetts Institute of Technology (MIT), used Rogers' therapy techniques to reflect back thoughts and feelings of the "patient" using rephrasing and repetition and stereotypical empathetic statements. Weizenbaum, who developed the program to show the limitations of artificial intelligence, was appalled that people took Eliza seriously as an alternative to face-to-face psychotherapy. In his book *Computers and Human Reason* (1976), he said that there are important differences between computers and human beings and that computers should and never could become psychotherapists.

At the present time we do not have completely convincing verbal psychotherapy that is generated by computers, but many think it is just a question of time before computers can approximate a therapist. Whether or not we will ever have completely automated interventions in suicide prevention that are comparable to, or can be used as a substitute for psychotherapy is still subject to debate. Some are still quite sceptical and we shall see in the coming years to what extent computerized therapy develops and becomes popular. Some may say that it would allow for more people to have access to psychotherapists if some problems could be simply handled by computer programs, thus leaving therapists to handle more complex difficulties. Perhaps psychotherapists will try to stop this from happening because it could potentially put them out of work. One thinks of Woody Allen's comedy routine in which he said "My father worked for the same firm for 12 years. They fired him and replaced him with a tiny gadget that does everything my father does – only better. The depressing thing is, my mother ran out and bought one too."

In the future we will see an increased use of automated programmes to identify people who are at risk of committing suicide, to make referrals to various services to obtain help and to provide some forms of preventive intervention. The use of artificial intelligence programs to mimic humans, for example by conducting follow-up calls or doing psychotherapy, is not a very creative way of using new technologies. It involves simply transforming human activities into automated computer programs. It is possible that in the future the tremendous processing power of computers will be used in new yet unheard-of ways which are unique to this media that will contribute to suicide prevention. It will be very interesting to see how things develop.

Research agenda

Research is needed to establish which interventions work, under what conditions, using which new technologies. We need to:

1. Demonstrate the use and effectiveness of using Internet services to provide crisis intervention, counselling, e-mail therapy, and all the other services that exist and will be developed in the near future. Research is needed to establish which services are effective in reaching suicidal persons who would otherwise not receive help, reaching people in suicidal crises and in helping to prevent suicides. Although this is extremely difficult to ascertain, it is paramount to the field of suicide prevention. We need to determine how many people and with which characteristics are effectively being referred to regular off-line help, how well series of repeated suicide attempts are interrupted, etc. This requires longitudinal research designs in which participants are followed over time, with all the associated practical

issues of maintaining contacts and ethical issues concerning what can constitute a control group condition and when to stop the research to intervene when participants may be at risk.

Once the effectiveness of services is determined, one could then perform cost-effectiveness analyses in order to demonstrate the cost savings of using new technologies when compared to traditional services.

2. Define target groups in the community that should be reached and helped by the new technologies and define research programmes that specifically establish the effectiveness of reaching and helping these groups. Once it has been determined that services have a positive impact on users, it is essential to determine if high risk target groups will actually use the services as planned. We must learn from research in other areas. For example, early campaigns to promote safe sex practices to prevent HIV/AIDS often found that the major impact in terms of behavioural changes had been with people who had a very low risk of exposure to HIV, but there was less impact on high risk groups. We need to determine if the target groups of people at risk of attempting suicide will actually use the interventions that have been proven to be effective.

3. Identify how to determine when suicide risk increases so that interventions can be targeted at the right people at the right time. New technologies have the potential of reaching suicidal people who are at the point of killing themselves. In order to do so, we must better understand how to identify when and how people proceed from suicidal thoughts and suicidal plans to the execution of their plans in a suicide attempt. We need to better understand this pre-suicidal process (or "syndrome") in detail to develop interventions that decelerate this process.

4. Demonstrate the incremental value of new technologies in improving the knowledge and skills of caregivers and gatekeepers. We need to determine the value of e-learning for teachers, mental health professionals, gatekeepers and others. If Internet e-learning is successfully evaluated and applied, there may be a substantial spread and increase in knowledge and skills in suicide prevention.

5. Assess the value of computerized identification of suicide risk for general practitioners, mental health professionals and workers in community agencies. If there is no advantage to using these automated devices, it is of no use to foster their use to replace clinical judgements. There even may be dangers involved: clinicians may

forget to ask the right questions while relying only on their computers in the next room, missing opportunities to build rapport and have more helpful interventions.

Methodological and ethical issues in Internet suicide prevention

Because of the great enthusiasm for the use of the Internet and other new technologies in suicide prevention, there are many *innovative but unproven* interventions being promoted. This is not a healthy state of affairs. Some over enthusiastic developers may be marketing Internet interventions that are not effective at all. One might think that when sufficient numbers of visitors use a particular service, that would be proof of its helpfulness. Unfortunately, that is not the case. There are many examples of unproven interventions that are not working and nonetheless attract many clients: homeopathic medicine, for example, or faith healers. Many innovative interventions may turn out to be very helpful, but one never can tell before they have been carefully tested.

The "gold standard" of research involves using a double-blind experimental design in which participants are randomly assigned to an experimental group that receives the new treatment or to a non-treatment control (comparison) group or a control group that receives "treatment as usual". In the area of suicide prevention, comparisons to a non-treatment group are generally considered unethical (Mishara and Weisstub, 2005). It is not considered ethical, and it is usually impossible to have proposals accepted by research ethics committees if the research involves identifying people as being at risk of suicide and not giving them any help because they were assigned to the control group. However, some of the new Internet interventions cannot be compared to treatment as usual, simply because there is no comparable treatment as usual. Simple before and after measurements can indicate the helpfulness of an intervention, as long as sufficient data are collected among completers and non-completers. However, one must compare interventions to determine if the treatment characteristics of the intervention are responsible for the positive outcomes or if other factors, such as simply giving any form of attention to people in need, would result in the same effects.

Research on the Internet of course has to deal with the issue of attrition. We know from studies of e-mental health and the few Internet interventions on suicidal ideation that have been evaluated that the likelihood of Internet users dropping out of research is much greater than in face-to-face interventions, particularly when participants are anonymous. This is not a problem generated by the research or the intervention; it reflects the natural tendency of people to drop out of anything that requires sustained attention on the Internet. This high rate of attrition renders some methodological requirements impossible to attain. When there are high attrition rates to be expected, one may not be able to confirm a significant impact of the treatment if the total sample that began the treatment is used in the analysis..

When including participants in research, it is a standard practice to obtain informed consent. However, participants who visit Internet sites often value their anonymity. When asked for informed consent, they have to disclose their identity and provide their signature. Because of this, many potential participants will not participate (see Chapter 4 in this book by Kerkhof et al.). The end result is that the group of respondents who are willing to give their consent may not be representative of users of the intervention, thus rendering the study less valuable. We therefore need thoughtful consideration from researchers as well as from ethics committees of whether in Internet studies informed consent can be possible while conserving anonymity. This is a fundamental issue. If this cannot be settled, many studies of the effectiveness of Internet interventions will not be possible.

When ethics committees evaluate research protocols on suicide prevention activities, they understandably point to the need for *safety plans* in case participants become acutely suicidal during the study. If the participants remain anonymous, the researchers cannot intervene if they learn that there is a risk of suicide or an attempt is in progress. Researchers can advise anonymous participants who become acutely suicidal to click on a button that will link or refer them to helplines or off-line crisis intervention services. People at risk of suicide who had not been involved in the research study would not have received such referrals, and may be at greater suicide risk for want of contact with resources to obtain help. We encourage researchers and ethics committees to carefully consider these issues and elaborate conditions under which Internet intervention studies could be carried out with anonymous participants.

This problem becomes all the more clear when it concerns young people. In order to study Internet interventions for suicidal screening and crisis intervention among youths, ethics committees generally require active informed consent from one, or sometimes from both parents. Not surprisingly, adolescents seldom ask their parents to sign a letter to obtain their permission to participate in a study of suicidal thinking and behaviour, particularly not when they are actually suicidal. This is an unfortunate state of affairs: a potential lifesaving intervention cannot be studied because of ethical restrictions. The end result is that the services provided to youths on the Internet will have to be provided without any quality guarantees and without the possibility that the effectiveness of these interventions can be studied scientifically with representative samples of users.

Another problem concerns the inclusion or exclusion of the most acutely suicidal persons who may need the Internet intervention most and may not use more traditional mental health and suicide prevention services. When acutely high risk individuals are excluded from evaluation research, the usefulness of the intervention to help those most in need may be impossible to assess. Many Internet interventions target the most acutely suicidal persons (e.g. billboards urging the use of their mobile phone for suicidal people standing at the side of a railway track). It would be odd to exclude these participants because of their high suicide risk. Furthermore, at a moment of acute suicidal crisis, it would be absurd to ask for informed consent to participate in the research study before proceeding to offer help.

There is a need to establish ethical guidelines as well as procedures for ethics committees to encompass the range of interventions using new technologies that allow for anonymity and provide help in acute crises, but without prior identification of the participants by signing the usual Consent Form which is generally required to conduct research with human participants. Furthermore, in the case of minors, where parental consent is usually required to participate in a research study, researchers will be blocked from assessing the impact of new Internet interventions for youths if signing traditional parental consent forms is a prerequisite to participating in the research study. The ethical basis of these practices needs to be clarified, and we need to develop a detailed code of ethics for studying interventions using new technologies in the 21st century.

We live in exciting times; we are on the frontier of the development of a wide range of new technologically advanced methods for preventing suicides. As the use of the Internet, smartphones and other technological advances become increasingly present, we are optimistic about their potential to save lives, prevent suicide attempts and help people bereaved by suicide. However, at the same time, we are also realistically cautious because of the paucity of research evaluations of the effectiveness of these new practices. There is a great gap between the development of services and the initiation of research programmes to determine which of these new services are effective and what constitutes the best practices using these new technologies. We look forward to learning much more to answer these questions in the coming years.

References

Marasinghe, R. H., Edirippulige, S., Kavanagh, D., Smith, A., & Jiffry, M. T. M. (2012). Effect of mobile phone-based psychotherapy in suicide prevention: A randomized controlled trial in Sri Lanka. *Journal of Telemedicine and Telecare, 18*(3), 151–155.

Mishara, B. L., & Weisstub, D. N. (2005). Ethical Issues in suicide research. *International Journal of Law and Psychiatry, 28*, 23–41.

Mishara, B. L., & Weisstub, D. N. (2007). Ethical, legal, and practical issues in the control and regulation of suicide promotion and assistance over the Internet. *Suicide and Life-Threatening Behavior, 37*(1), 58–65.

Mishara, B. L., & Weisstub, D. N. (2010). Resolving ethical dilemmas in suicide prevention: The case of telephone helpline rescue policies. *Suicide and Life-Threatening Behavior, 40*(2), 159–169.

Stanley, B., & Brown, G. K. (2012). Safety planning intervention: A brief intervention to mitigate suicide risk. *Cognitive and Behavioural Practice, 19*, 256–264.

Weizenbaum, J.(1976). *Computer and human reason: From judgment to calculation.* San Francisco, CA: W.H. Freeman and Company.

Index

MAR 2 6 2014

Printed and bound in the United States of America